Suggested citation

Moriyama IM, Loy RM, Robb-Smith AHT. History of the statistical classification of diseases and causes of death. Rosenberg HM, Hoyert DL, eds. Hyattsville, MD: National Center for Health Statistics. 2011.

Library of Congress Cataloging-in-Publication Data

Moriyama, Iwao M. (Iwao Milton), 1909-2006, author.
History of he sta is ical classification of diseases and causes of death / by Iwao M. Moriyama, Ph.D., Ruth M. Loy, MBE, A.H.T. Robb-Smith, M.D. ; edited and updated by Harry M. Rosenberg, Ph.D., Donna L. Hoyert, Ph.D.
    p. ; cm. -- (DHHS publication ; no. (PHS) 2011-1125)
    "March 2011."
    Includes bibliographical references.

1. Interna ional sta is ical classification of diseases and related health problems. 10th revision. 2. International statistical classification of diseases and related health problems. 11th revision. 3. Nosology--History. 4. Death--Causes--Classification--History. I. Loy, Ruth M., author. II. Robb-Smith, A. H. T. (Alastair Hamish Tearloch), author. III. Rosenberg, Harry M. (Harry Michael), editor. IV. Hoyert, Donna L., editor. V. National Center for Health Sta is ics (U.S.) VI. Title. VII. Series: DHHS publica ion ; no. (PHS) 2011-1125.
    [DNLM: 1. International classification of diseases. 2. Disease--classification. 3. International Classification of Diseases--history. 4. Cause of Death. 5. History, 20th Century. WB 15]
    RB115.M72 2011
    616.07'8012--dc22

    2010044437

For sale by the U.S. Government Printing Office
Superintendent of Documents
Mail Stop: SSOP
Washington, DC 20402–9328
Printed on acid-free paper.

History of the Statistical Classification of Diseases and Causes of Death

Iwao M. Moriyama, Ph.D.
Ruth M. Loy, M.B.E.
Alastair H.T. Robb-Smith, M.D.

Edited and updated by
Harry M. Rosenberg, Ph.D.
Donna L. Hoyert, Ph.D.

2011

National Center for Health Statistics

Edward J. Sondik, Ph.D., *Director*
Jennifer H. Madans, Ph.D., *Associate Director for Science*

Division of Vital Statistics

Charles J. Rothwell, M.S., *Director*

DEDICATION

Dr. Iwao M. Moriyama wished to dedicate this report to the memory of Dr. Halbert L. Dunn (1896–1975), whom he described as a man "whose visions became a reality at the Sixth Decennial Revision Conference" at Palais D'Orsay in Paris on April 30, 1948. Dr. Moriyama (1909–2006) directly participated in many of the 20th century developments described in this report, at the same time taking on a succession of positions and responsibilities between 1940 and 1975 within what ultimately became the National Center for Health Statistics. Following his retirement from federal service, Dr. Moriyama continued to have a significant role in the vital statistics community as director of the International Institute for Vital Registration and Statistics. Throughout his life, Dr. Moriyama continued to challenge his successors to achieve best practices for mortality statistics.

Edward J. Sondik, Ph.D.
Director
National Center for Health Statistics

March 2011

ABOUT THE AUTHORS

Iwao M. Moriyama, M.P.H., Ph.D.

Executive Director, International Institute for Vital Registration and Statistics

Associate Director for International Statistics, National Center for Health Statistics, 1974–1975

Director, Office of Health Statistics Analysis, National Center for Health Statistics, 1961–1974

Head, U.S. Delegation to the International Conference for the Ninth Decennial Revision of the International Classification of Diseases (ICD), 1975

Member, U.S. Delegation to the International Conference for the Decennial Revision of the ICD, Sixth to Ninth Revisions

Member, Expert Committee on Classification of Diseases, World Health Organization (WHO), 1947–1975

Executive Secretary, U.S. National Committee on Vital and Health Statistics, 1949–1975

Member, Advisory Committee for Current Medical Terminology, American Medical Association, 1963–1968

Ruth M. Loy, M.B.E.

Senior Executive Officer, WHO Collaborating Center for Classification of Diseases, London (retired 1982)

WHO Collaborating Center for Classification of Diseases, London, 1966–1982

Assisted WHO Secretariat on Classification of Diseases at WHO meetings of Heads of Collaborating Centers on Disease Classification, Expert Committee meetings on disease classification

Conducted WHO training courses for reorientation of coders upon introduction of Eighth and Ninth Revisions of the ICD

Alastair H.T. Robb-Smith, M.A., M.D., F.R.C.P.

Consultant pathologist and former Director of Pathology, United Oxford Hospitals (England)

Emeritus Nuffield Reader in Pathology, University of Oxford

Editor, Medical Research Council's *A Provisional Classification of Diseases and Injuries for Use in Compiling Morbidity Statistics*, 1944

Member, Nomenclature of Diseases Committee, Royal College of Physicians, 1948–1969

Member, Expert Committee on Classification of Diseases, WHO, 1947–1970

Chairman, Registrar-General's Advisory Committee for the Eighth Revision of the ICD, 1961–1965

Member, U.K. Delegation to the Eighth Decennial Revision Conference, Geneva, 1965

Chairman, Committee on Disease Nomenclature, Council for International Organizations of Medical Sciences, 1968

Contents

Foreword

This report describes the historic development of the disease nomenclatures and classifications that ultimately became the major international standard known as the World Health Organization's (WHO) International Classification of Diseases (ICD). Written largely at the initiative of Dr. Iwao Moriyama, a participant in these developments for much of the 20th century, the report describes the historical, cultural, and scientific environment in which ICD evolved, expanded, and improved. Although the report focuses on the application of ICD to mortality, it also touches on nonmortality applications, particularly as these affected the classification for mortality.

With respect to mortality, the report is broad in scope. It begins by briefly describing the registration system used to collect death data, including cause of death (Chapter 1), and notes periodic efforts to standardize language that might be used to convey information in the death registration system (Chapter 2), but focuses on the classification, how the language reported in the registration system is collapsed into this classification (Chapter 3), and other issues associated with the classification's development (Chapter 4). The report discusses issues, some singular and some recurrent, that needed to be addressed during the evolution of ICD (Chapters 4 and 8), and describes the expanding application of the classification from a narrow focus on causes of death to the broader scope of causes of illness, and from an emphasis on statistical presentation and analysis to administrative uses such as hospital records indexing and medical billing (Chapter 7). The report also discusses implications of ICD choices on quality and statistics (Chapters 5 and 6).

The history of ICD is rich in international collaboration and cooperation. This, and the fact that it is a classification based on sound, time-tested principles, accounts for its long and continuous international acceptance. More use is now being made of ICD than ever before. To meet

Lasker Group Award
Presented to the U.S. Committee on Joint Causes of Death, 1947

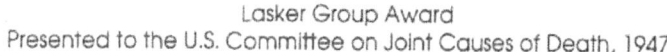

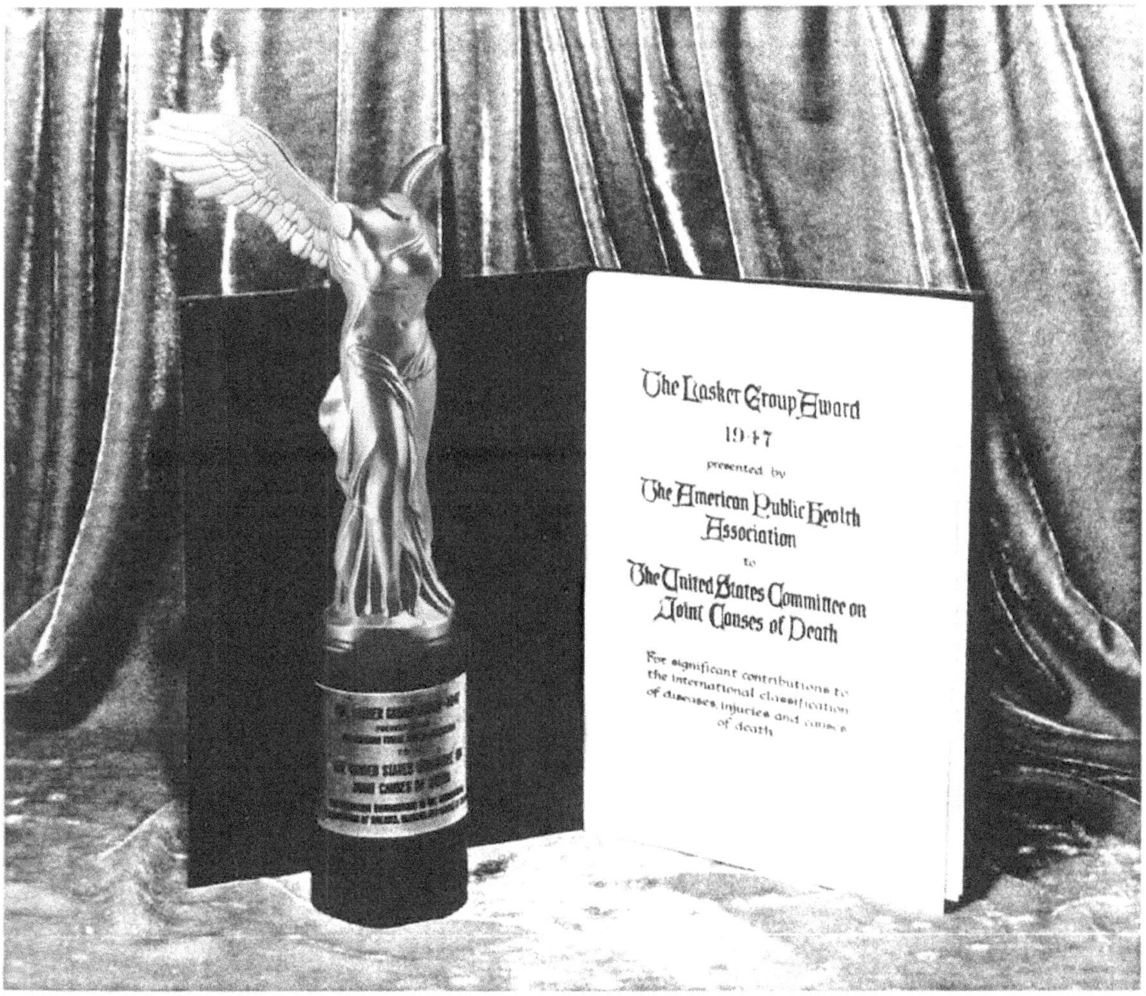

| ix |

the demands for greater detail in disease classification, ICD has greatly expanded in successive revisions; this expansion can be expected to continue as the nonstatistical uses of ICD grow. This history of ICD is intended to help provide perspective as ICD continues to evolve in response to changing medical, social, and technological imperatives.

The development and continuing evolution of ICD reflects the untiring efforts of many people. William Farr, Marc d'Espine, and Jacques Bertillon have been credited as the founders of ICD. Bertillon led the preparations for the initial decennial revisions of the *International Lists of Causes of Death*. Many others have contributed to preparatory work, guidance, and oversight in subsequent revisions, including Dr. Knud Stouman of the Health Section of the League of Nations; Dr. Marie Cakrtova, Dr. Karel Kupka, Graham Corbett, Andre L'Hours, and Dr. Gerlind Bamer of WHO; members of the WHO Expert Committees on Health Statistics; and the WHO Collaborating Centers for the Family of International Classifications. Other individuals had major involvement in ICD-related activities, such as studies on joint causes of death that led to adopting the concept of the underlying cause of death, and significant work done to implement this decision. These included Dr. Halbert L. Dunn, Chief, Vital Statistics Division, U.S. Bureau of the Census and head of the U.S. Delegation to the Fifth Revision Conference; and a subcommittee of the U.S. Committee on Joint Causes of Death comprising Dr. Percy Stocks, Medical Statistician of the General Register Office of England and Wales; Dr. Alastair H.T. Robb-Smith, Pathologist, Radcliffe Infirmary, Oxford University; Winifred O'Brien, Nosologist, Dominion Bureau of Statistics, Canada; Dr. W. Thurber Fales, Statistician, Baltimore City Health Department; Dr. Selwyn D. Collins, Statistician, U.S. Public Health Service; and Dr. Iwao M. Moriyama, Statistician, U.S. Bureau of the Census.

A few of these many important contributions have been recognized. For example, Farr, d'Espine, and Bertillon were memorialized at the commemoration of the centenary of ICD on September 7, 1994, at the Palais de Nation in Geneva, Switzerland. In 1947, the American Public Health Association presented the U.S. Committee on Joint Causes of Death with the Lasker Group Award (see photo) for the work that led to adoption of the underlying cause concept.

Two coauthors of the present report, Moriyama and Robb-Smith, became associated with the ICD revision process at the preparatory stage of the Sixth Revision and worked on subsequent revisions through the Ninth Revision. The third coauthor, Loy, assisted the WHO Secretariat starting with the Eighth Revision and continuing into the Tenth Revision. Consequently, the text is enhanced by the authors' personal knowledge and involvement in many of the 20th century developments described.

For preparing this report, the International Statistical Institute, WHO, the United Kingdom's Office of National Statistics, and the National Center for Health Statistics (NCHS) provided free access to documents and publications dealing with ICD. From NCHS, A. Joan Klebba and Mabel Smith were particularly helpful in searching for and providing revisions of the medical certificate forms and the lists of causes of death. Dr. Michael A. Heasman, Dr. Josephine Weatherall, Dr. Paul M. Densen, Robert A. Israel, and Alice B. Dolman provided helpful comments on various drafts of this history. Lillian Guralnick and Mary Anne Freedman provided editorial assistance. Dr. David Berglund provided helpful comments on the discussion of the *Systematized Nomenclature of Medicine*. Dr. Harry M. Rosenberg extensively edited and updated the entire report to reflect recent developments in ICD, technology applications to mortality, and policy implications of recent ICD revisions. Finally, Dr. Donna L. Hoyert ushered the report through the final stages of the publication process, including responding to reviewer comments and inserting additional updates.

| x |

CHAPTER 1

Evolution of Death Registration

To produce statistics on causes of illness and causes of death, parallel sets of information are needed: for illnesses, a source of morbidity data, a classification of diseases, and guidelines for designating a principal condition from among several that may be listed on a medical record; and for deaths, some form of death report, a disease classification, and a set of rules for selecting a single cause of death for each decedent.

In the case of statistics on cause of death, the origins of two of these prerequisites, death registration and disease classification, are closely interrelated both historically and intellectually. Concerns about recurrent epidemics and their prevention, scientific advancement, and political reorganization stimulated the organization of public health, including the registration of deaths and classification of their causes. This chapter traces the evolution of death registration and the form of death report or certificate used in the registration process in the United States and internationally. Chapter 4 focuses on the third prerequisite, cause of death, the condition of most relevance for statistical and analytical uses.

Origins of death registration

The beginnings of death registration can be found in mid-15th century Italy, where medical education and social administration were more advanced than elsewhere in Europe. The Councilors for the cities of northern Italy, remembering the great pandemics of plague in the century before that killed more than one-third of the whole population of Europe, set up boards of health to consider how best to deal with the recurring epidemics that ravaged their populations. These boards of health enjoyed considerable power, but they were essentially administrative and autocratic in nature. Although the detailed practices of the board of one city might differ a little from those of another, the basic principles under which they operated were fairly uniform. For example, a death certificate or bill of mortality was required to be filed, containing the name and age of the deceased and the cause of death certified by a physician or a certified surgeon, before a burial certificate could be issued and

arrangements could be made. In many of the cities, the volumes containing these certificates dating to the 15th century are still preserved.

Extending from this were quarantine regulations, that is, restriction of movement without license and supervision of sanitary conditions in dwellings and in facilities for people who were infected (i.e., pesthouses). Although the causes of infection were unknown, edicts were issued that required fumigation where death had taken place. At one time, all cats and dogs were ordered destroyed, increasing the rat population. The boards of health were also authorized to deal with the quality of foods and water and the disposal of refuse and sewage. Another advantage of the boards' administrative structure was the transmission of information about diseases from one city to another and about epidemic occurrences in other countries, which ambassadors to those countries conveyed.

In the 16th century, boards of health were set up in France, Switzerland, and the Netherlands, but they were only temporary measures during a crisis, not continuous organizations as in Italy. The practice of requiring a death certificate before a burial permit could be issued spread from the Italian boards of health to other European countries over time. Because they contained the name and age of the decedent and the cause of death, data from the death certificates were used to monitor epidemics in the various cities.

In England, three activities that foreshadowed death registration began in the 1530s: 1) In 1532, one of the earliest, if not the earliest, systematic collection of data on causes of death, the Bills of Mortality, began. These weekly lists of burials in London included the name of the deceased, the parish in which the burial took place, and the cause of death, with particular reference to the plague. The cause of death was determined by searchers, or "wise women" as they were known, after they had viewed the body. In more difficult cases, the searcher consulted a physician. The searchers made their reports to the parish clerk, who prepared an account of all burials in the preceding week every Tuesday night. In these accounts, the numbers of deaths from plague and all other causes were summed at the end of the listing. On Wednesdays, the general account was made and printed. The bills were distributed on Thursday to subscribers who paid 4 shillings for an annual subscription. 2) In 1534, Queen Elizabeth introduced quarantine and plague orders in England. 3) Shortly thereafter, parish registers were also established in England. These registers recorded baptisms rather than births and burials instead of deaths, and the registers contained no information on causes of death.

More than a century later, John Graunt conceived of the idea of using the Bills of Mortality for analytical purposes (1). He made ingenious use of imperfect data and made a number of generalizations, such as mortality in the earliest years of life being relatively high. In the absence of mortality data by age, Graunt estimated the number of deaths among children under age 5 years as follows: "Having premised these general Advertisements, our first observations upon the Casualties shall be, that in twenty years there dying of all Diseases and Casualties, 229,150 that 71,124 dyed of the Thrush, Convulsions, Rickets, Teeth, and Worms; and as Abortives, Chrysomes, Infants, Livergrowns, and Overlaids; that is to say, that about 1/3 of the whole dies of those Diseases, which we guess did all light upon children under four or five years old" (1).

Despite medical progress, the diagnostic quality of the bills did not improve. Interest in these bills also waned. Clerks of many parishes failed to report or reported only irregularly. Even when complete, the Bills of Mortality gave no information about the population much beyond the walls of London.

Starting in the mid-18th century, national civil registration systems came into being and made possible the continuous recording of births and deaths and the annual compilation of birth and death statistics. However, it was not yet possible to produce comparable statistics on causes of death as disease classification had not reached that stage of development (see Chapter 3).

In 1837, the Registration Act was passed in England with provisions for inquiry into causes of death in the population. In 1839, William Farr was appointed compiler of abstracts in the Registrar-General's office, and he, probably more than anyone else, developed and analyzed mortality statistics to delineate the sanitary and health problems of the day (2,3). After Florence Nightingale returned to England from the Crimean War, she promoted the importance of and the need for hospital data and statistics on causes of illness and causes of death in the armed forces at the political level, and she enlisted the aid of Farr to work on the technical aspects of these problems.

Death registration in the United States

The English Registration Act of 1837 served as the prototype of the first state registration law in the United States, enacted by Massachusetts in 1842. In the years following, births and deaths were registered in a few of the largest cities and several states. In 1855, the American Medical Association (AMA) adopted a resolution urging its members to take immediate and concerted action in petitioning legislative bodies to establish offices for the registration of vital events. By 1900, 10 states and the District of Columbia had met the requirements of the U.S. Bureau of the Census for admission to the U.S. Death Registration Area. The compilation of annual mortality statistics for the United States began with these states in 1900. Nationwide coverage was achieved in 1933.

Unlike most countries, the civil registration system in the United States is a decentralized system, that is, responsibility for the registration of vital events is in the hands of the individual states (4). There is no national registration office—states have complete autonomy with respect to registration matters. The system is coordinated by the Centers for Disease Control and Prevention's (CDC) National Center for Health Statistics (NCHS). Within NCHS, the Division of Vital Statistics is responsible for setting standards and guidelines that have generally been accepted voluntarily by state offices, and for the national compilation of vital statistics.

In most countries except the United States, a family member or relative is required to appear before the local registrar to register the death. The local registrar records certain personal particulars and information about the death. If the registration law calls for data on causes of death, the hospital in which the death took place or the physician in attendance is required to forward the information to the local registrar.

In the United States, the funeral director, not the family member, is responsible for notifying the local registrar of the death. He or she obtains from a family member the personal particulars of the decedent and other information called for on the death certificate. He or she also obtains from the physician in attendance at death a completed and duly signed medical certificate of death. If the death occurred without medical attention or resulting from violence or suspected foul play, the case is referred to the medicolegal authority, a coroner or medical examiner appointed locally, for review or investigation.

The death certificate that the registrar files in the United States is a combined legal and statistical form that includes the medical certificate of cause of death. Upon filing the death certificate with the local registrar, the funeral director receives a burial permit or a burial transit permit if the remains are to be shipped to another state.

While registration practices differ somewhat by country, official mortality statistics on causes of death are generally derived from the death record filed in compliance with the registration law to prevent the illegal disposition of human remains. Cause-of-death statistics are mainly by-products of a legal process, the registration of death. However, not all countries are able to produce cause-of-death statistics using the registration model, for example, because their medical care system does not extend to a large part of the population. A later chapter examines lay reporting of causes of death as an alternative source of data (Chapter 4). A classification of diseases provides a method for the medical information reported in a registration system to be organized to facilitate producing and using statistics; development of this classification is discussed beginning in Chapter 3.

| 3 |

CHAPTER 2

Nomenclature of Diseases

For precision in reporting causes of illness or death, a nomenclature of diseases is essential. A nomenclature is a list of acceptable or approved disease terminology and differs from a classification, which refers to disease terms organized in a systematic way. Many disease nomenclatures are listings of diseases in alphabetical order. Such a simple alphabetic arrangement of disease terms is not regarded as a disease classification. However, when the disease terms are grouped according to topographic site and etiology, they become disease classifications. The semantic distinction between the terms "nomenclature" and "classification" has not always been maintained in use. For example, the first Bertillon classification in 1899, predecessor to the *International Classification of Diseases* (ICD), was called a nomenclature even though it was designed to be a statistical classification.

This chapter reviews initiatives, both in the United States and internationally, to develop nomenclatures for diseases and medical procedures, a process related to and paralleling efforts to develop a classification of diseases for statistical purposes. Although clarity and precision might be enhanced if a nomenclature was used in reporting cause of death in death registration, death registration has developed solutions to accommodate the variety of terms actually reported on a death certificate. Use of the classification is described in Chapter 3.

Need for nomenclature

In the first Annual Report of the Registrar-General of England and Wales in 1839, Farr said, "The advantages of a uniform nomenclature, however imperfect, are so obvious, that it is surprising no attention has been paid to its enforcement in Bills of Mortality. Each disease has, in many instances, been denoted by three or four terms, and each term has been applied to as many different diseases: vague, inconvenient names have been employed, or complications have been registered instead of primary diseases. The nomenclature is of as much importance in this department of enquiry as weights and measures in the physical sciences, and should be settled without delay" (5).

The purpose of a disease nomenclature is to promote the use of the most appropriate diagnostic term to describe a particular disease. A generally accepted standard or authoritative medical vocabulary comprised of unambiguous medical terminology is essential for precise and effective communication about disease and medical entities. The recorded diagnostic information should convey accurately and completely the description of diseases as observed by the clinician. To serve its full function, a medical nomenclature should be extensive, so that any morbid or pathological condition that can be accurately and specifically described has a place.

Most disease nomenclatures of the past have included only recommended or acceptable terminology. However, limiting the disease nomenclature to acceptable terminology does not always achieve the objective of uniformity in the use of diagnostic terms. If the clinician does not know the precise diagnostic term but knows the disease by its eponym or by some other term (synonyms or otherwise), he or she is not able to find that disease term in any list of acceptable medical terminology without a good deal of trial and error. Even so, he or she may have come up with a term that is not exactly the same as the disease under discourse. Thus, an alphabetic index of a disease nomenclature should include synonyms, eponyms, and other equivalents even though they are not considered proper terminology. All of these terms can be cross-referenced to the "approved" term, with preferred terms so designated.

Development of disease terminology

The first authoritative source of disease terminology dates to the mid-19th century when the Royal College of Physicians published its nomenclature of disease (6,7). This was followed shortly by the AMA's nomenclature of disease and subsequently by other efforts (8,9).

Early in 1857, the Hospital Committee of the Epidemiological Society of London decided a new nomenclature of diseases was needed to achieve uniformity in the mode of recording diseases and thus facilitating statistical and other enquiries, an idea already advocated by *The Lancet* and by Sir David Dumbreck, Inspector-General of Military Hospitals. The committee then wrote to the Royal College of Physicians, stating that the Epidemiological Society and the Directors-General of the Army and Navy, East India Company, and Metropolitan Hospitals had agreed to draw up a nomenclature of diseases for common use in those organizations. Farr was to act for the Registrar-General, and the presidents of the College of Physicians and Surgeons had sanctioned the project. The committee believed these aims could best be achieved if the college was responsible for preparing the nomenclature (6,7).

The committee started to meet fortnightly in late 1857. Some 12 years later, the long-awaited *Nomenclature of Diseases, Presented by the Royal College of Physicians of London* was published. It was a listing of approved names of diseases in English, Latin, German, French, and Italian, together with synonyms of the English names and, in many cases, definitions. The sequential arrangement was essentially anatomical.

The layout and indexes were easily understood, and the foreword emphasized that this was essentially a nosological [i.e., having to do with the "branch of medical science that deals with the classification of diseases" (10)] grouping, not a classification. The note was presumably made to forestall the objections of the Registrar-General, who was concerned that the *Nomenclature of Diseases* might be used as a weapon to strengthen the hand of the British Medical Association and the Medical Officers of the Health Association to take on the National Registration of Disease.

The *Nomenclature of Diseases, Presented by the Royal College of Physicians* was revised from time to time (1885, 1896, 1906, 1918, 1931, 1947, and the ninth, or last, edition in 1959) to provide an authoritative source of medical terminology for British physicians. After the initial edition, the nomenclature evolved into a list of preferred terms in English without definition. At the anniversary dinner held at the college in 1969, the president announced that, after consultation with interested bodies, it had been decided to cease publication of the nomenclature. However, the college would always collaborate in any matter concerned with the nomenclature or the classification of diseases (6,7).

In 1869, the Surgeon General of the U.S. Army had called to the AMA's attention the disease nomenclature of the Royal College of Physicians and suggested that it be used by American physicians. An AMA committee considered the proposal and concluded that it would be better for AMA to draw up an American nomenclature. In 1872, AMA published its *Nomenclature of Diseases*. However,

this activity was soon discontinued (8).

In 1908, Cressy Wilbur, Chief of the Division of Vital Statistics, U.S. Bureau of the Census, persuaded AMA to set up a committee on nomenclature and classification of disease, and recommended that the 1909 conference for the revision of the *International List of Causes of Death* also take up the problem of an international nomenclature of diseases and injuries with precise agreement on the meaning of terms (11). To achieve this end, Wilbur approached the Royal College of Physicians for its support. The college was already working on the fifth revision of its nomenclature and showed little enthusiasm to get involved in the preparation of an international nomenclature. World War I intervened, and it became apparent that an enterprise of this magnitude could not be undertaken under war conditions. The AMA committee was therefore discharged.

During the war, the need for a uniform nomenclature could no longer be avoided, and steps were taken that resulted in the 1919 publication of the *Standard Nomenclature of Diseases and Pathological Conditions, Injuries and Poisonings for the United States* by the U.S. Bureau of the Census (11). It was based on the eight nomenclatures then in use, but because it consisted of only an alphabetical list of names with code numbers, it had very little use or influence.

Although no single set of acceptable medical terminology existed in the United States, some large hospitals like Bellevue and Allied Hospitals in New York City, Massachusetts General Hospital in Boston, and Johns Hopkins University Hospital in Baltimore had their own medical nomenclature. In 1928, the New York Academy of Medicine, at the suggestion of George Baehr, called a National Conference on Nomenclature of Disease to which the principal medical societies, the armed services, hospitals, and public health organizations were invited. The conference decided to undertake preparing a standard nomenclature of diseases with H.P. Logie as Executive Secretary (9). The basic plan for the nomenclature was adopted in 1930, and the first publication appeared in 1932, the First Revision in 1933, and the Second Edition in 1935. In 1937, AMA took over responsibility for the periodic revisions. The revision that appeared in 1942 also included a standard nomenclature of operations (8).

The *Standard Nomenclature of Diseases and Operations* (SNDO) underwent several revisions, the last in 1961 (8). After the Fifth Edition was issued, AMA decided to abandon it. SNDO provided a list of acceptable diagnostic terminology, but because the terms lacked definition, SNDO was found not particularly useful as a disease nomenclature. SNDO's complete specificity, making it a less efficient instrument for the retrieval of hospital records for clinical study, clinched the argument for discontinuing its publication and issuing instead *Current Medical*

Terminology (12–14). However, continued use was made of SNDO for indexing medical records until a more efficient method was found.

The First Edition of *Current Medical Terminology* was published in 1963 as a medical dictionary with an alphabetical index of preferred terms. The Second Edition, issued in 1964, was devised for use in standardizing disease terminology for medical records, communication, and computer analysis. The Fourth Edition was retitled *Current Medical Information and Terminology* (CMIT). The Fifth Edition was published in 1981.

These terminologies are structured as follows: The preferred term is followed by one or two 2-digit code numbers. The 2-digit system designation is followed by a random 4-digit identification number that also appears on the first line of each entry. For each preferred term, the entries are:

■ Additional terms, including synonyms and eponyms

■ Etiologies designating or suggesting causes of the disease

■ Symptoms or complaints of the patient

■ Physical signs, including mental status findings, observed on examination or during patient interview

■ Laboratory data, including special tests and examinations such as EEG, ECG, ophthalmoscopy, and endoscopy

■ Pertinent radiological findings

■ Disease course and prognosis, including complications and results of treatment when known

■ Pathological findings, including gross and microscopic findings

A supplemental index, divided into main sections according to an alphabetized body system classification, offers guidance on selecting the preferred terms to describe diseases primarily associated with a specific body system. A numeric index of CMIT identification numbers is provided for computer application. One problem with a simple listing of disease terms in a nomenclature is that the meaning of any term may not be clear; to overcome this, CMIT includes signs and symptoms, etiology, complications, pathology, and laboratory findings, including X-rays—in effect, the diagnostic criteria for recording a diagnosis.

To be useful, a medical terminology must be continually updated. As new diagnostic terms are described, the nomenclature must accommodate them. Conversely, as medical knowledge increases and certain diagnostic

terms become obsolete, they must be replaced in the nomenclature by more precise terms.

A companion volume to *Current Medical Terminology* that dealt with medical procedures appeared in 1966 as *Current Procedural Terminology* (CPT) (15) and is now in its Fourth Edition (16). CPT–4 is a listing of descriptive terms and identifying codes for reporting medical services and procedures performed by physicians. It provides uniformity in communication among physicians, patients, and third parties.

While nothing came of Wilbur's proposal to prepare an international nomenclature of diseases in anticipation of the Second Decennial Conference for the Revision of the International List of Causes of Death, some 60 years later the Council for International Organizations of Medical Sciences (CIOMS), in a joint project with the World Health Organization (WHO), set about to prepare the *International Nomenclature of Diseases* (IND), which could be related to ICD (7). IND's purpose was to provide a single recommended name for every disease entity. The main criteria for selection of that name were that it should be specific, unambiguous, as self-descriptive and simple as possible, and based on cause wherever feasible. Each disease or syndrome for which a name was recommended was defined as unambiguously and yet as briefly as possible. A list of synonyms is appended to each definition.

At the Tenth Revision Conference of the International Classification of Diseases held in 1989 (17), it was reported that CIOMS had published the volumes on diseases of the lower respiratory tract, infectious diseases (viral, bacterial, and parasitic diseases, and mycoses) and cardiac and vascular diseases, and that work was under way on volumes for the digestive system, female genital system, metabolic and endocrine diseases, blood and blood-forming organs, immunological system, musculoskeletal system, and nervous system. Subjects proposed for future volumes included psychiatric diseases, as well as diseases of the skin, ear, nose, and throat, and eye and adnexa.

A more recent and ongoing related development, the *Systematized Nomenclature of Medicine*, is discussed in Chapter 7.

| 7 |

Development of the Classification of Diseases

To produce comparable cause-of-death statistics, development of a disease classification was needed so that information collected in death registration could be grouped and displayed in a similar way in different places. The great enthusiasm for organizing knowledge using a variety of taxonomic schemes, applied to nature and ideas in the 18th century and to Farr's work in England in the 19th century, stimulated continuing international initiatives on the classification of diseases that laid the groundwork for ICD. This chapter describes the development of the classification of diseases, its formal endorsement as an international standard by the late 19th century, and its further evolution, through successive revisions, to the present Tenth Revision (ICD–10). The chapter concludes with a discussion of WHO's continuous updating process, introduced with ICD–10.

Early disease classifications

In 15th century Italy, the disease classification used by physicians was largely based philosophically on humoral theories of disease, with occasional suggestions that malign outside influences might cause illness or death. Diseases were grouped in relation to these theories in the hope that this might throw light on their nature and possible treatment, but classifications based on these theories were of little assistance in the understanding of disease and the disease process.

In the 18th century, diseases captured the attention of those determined to organize knowledge, establish orderly groupings of natural objects, and develop encyclopedias. Although some groupings of diseases were evident in the early writings of the Greeks and Romans, the first serious attempt to develop a comprehensive approach to the classification of disease is found in Jean Fernel's *Universa Medicini* published in 1554, followed in 1685 by Thomas Sydenham's *Opera Omnia*.

A complete or at least very considerable change in the approach to the classification of diseases took place in the 18th century after a number of physicians such as F. Boissier de la Croix de Sauvages, Carolus Linnaeus, and later Erasmus Darwin and Jean-Louis Marc Alibert (who were also botanists) became interested in disease classifications. As plants were being divided and subdivided into various categories, so a similar system was adopted by Sauvages and others for classifying diseases. For example, Sauvages' comprehensive treatise, published under the title *Nosologia Methodica,* had 10 classes, mainly symptoms that were subdivided into some 300 orders and subdivided again into genera. That was followed by the division between "natural" and "artificial" systems. The artificial system took one particular manifestation of a disease as the feature on which classifications should be built, whereas the natural system required a large number of manifestations before two conditions were grouped together.

By the mid-18th century, the importance of morbid anatomy became apparent when it was recognized that many diseases could affect particular organs. This made a morphological classification dealing with these diseases acceptable and useful. The beginning of an understanding of epidemic diseases as derived from outside sources was taking hold, although the connection was still not very clear.

In 1775, William Cullen's *Synopsis Nosologae Methodicae* appeared (18). Although he was loud in his criticism of his predecessors, his categories were largely symptomatic and, as Farr later pointed out, the arrangements could not be used for statistical analysis.

In 1817, two books were published: Alibert's *Nosologie Naturelle,* the last of the old "botanical" systems of nosology, and John Mason Good's *A Physiological System of Nosology*. Good's classification, a new approach, was incorporated into his textbook of medicine and was the pattern for future medical textbooks. Although it had little influence on the statistical classification of diseases, it formed a basis for development of disease nomenclatures.

William Farr's classification

In 1839, Farr called attention to the importance of a uniform statistical classification of causes of death; his first attempt at a disease classification for statistical purposes appeared in the *First Annual Report of the Registrar-General of Births, Deaths, and Marriages* in England (2,3). After considering all the nosologies that existed at the time, Farr concluded that *Nosologia Methodica* by Sauvages was the first important work of its kind, noting that a number of his successors such as Linnaeus and Darwin had made comparatively few innovations or improvements. Farr suggested that Sauvages' system would have been adopted more widely if not for Cullen, whose nosology became established in Great Britain because of the simplicity and merits of its classification but also because of Cullen's popularity as a teacher and writer.

Although Cullen's nosology was in general use in the public services, Farr pointed out that pathological anatomy had progressed a great deal since Cullen's time and concluded that his classification no longer presented diseases in their "presumed natural relations." Farr also decided that the existing classification, an alphabetic listing starting with "abortives" and ending with "worms," was not satisfactory. He then considered various nosologies, testing among others those of Good and Cullen, and concluded that most classifications were too detailed for statistical use. Farr was interested in making statistical inferences and believed this could not be done from the small numbers that would result from a detailed classification. For this reason, he also did not provide specific rubrics for diseases that were rare in England.

Farr put forward an eclectic system based on the way diseases affect the population. He divided these into three classes, the first for those that occur endemically or epidemically, in other words, the communicable diseases, which provided an index of salubrity. The second class was for those diseases that arise sporadically—these he subdivided anatomically into diseases of the nervous system, respiratory organs, etc., ending with a group for those of uncertain location such as tumors, malformations, debility, sudden death, and old age. In each anatomical group, he characterized the more common conditions, ending with a residual category for the less common or ill-defined conditions. His third group was for death by violence. Farr emphasized that no classification could be successful unless a uniform and precise nomenclature was adopted that "would preclude the same disease being designated by four or five different names, or ambiguous terms being employed denoting no distinct malady, or applying popularly to several maladies." Farr's nosology was employed for more than 20 years by the General Register Office for England and Wales for its classification of causes of death. He was familiar with the practical problems of applying his classification to the medical certificates being filed in England and Wales.

Farr did much to promote his classification but could not find general acceptance. For example, Marc d'Espine of Geneva questioned his class of disease referable to various organ systems because this would fragment counts of diseases like tuberculosis and syphilis into various anatomic sites. Others were unable to accept Farr's notion of epidemic, endemic, and contagious diseases. Farr made some concessions to his critics, but the general framework of his classification remained unchanged. For a detailed discussion of Farr's statistical nosology, see Pelling (3) and Eyler (2).

First International Classification of Diseases

The triggering event leading to development of the first ICD was the unlikely Great Exhibition of 1851 held at the Crystal Palace in London. There, many nations displayed their industrial products, engendering a general air of excitement among visiting statisticians and other learned people over the idea of comparing statistically not only the quantity, but also the quality and other characteristics, of the industrial output of goods. These ideas stimulated the calling of the First International Statistical Congress at Brussels in 1853. By this time, a systematic review seems to have occurred of subjects that could be candidates for international statistical comparison, for one of the topics considered was "Causes of Death." Up to this point, statistics on causes of deaths were published for only a small number of countries; variations in the way diseases and accidents were described necessitated a uniform nomenclature and classification applicable to all countries.

Achille Guillard, a distinguished botanist and statistician, put forward a resolution for preliminary studies for a uniform nomenclature, to be discussed at a later congress (Guillard was later described as the creator not only of the science of demography but of the term "demography"). From 1853, the congress met approximately every two years until 1878. It was succeeded in 1885 by the biennial meetings of the International Statistical Institute (ISI), which continue to this day.

At the First Congress, lively discussions of the proposal took place, including presentation of the view that a uniform list was impossible because of the different training of doctors and their tendency to call diseases by whatever name they chose. The prevailing belief was that it should be possible to devise a list of diseases to which doctors would adhere, resulting in comparable statistics. It was recognized that advances in medical knowledge would make changes necessary from time to time.

D'Espine and Farr were charged with the task of drafting the list that would be applicable to all countries, marking the beginning of a long history of international collaboration to develop a uniform classification. They could not agree on the basis of the list and presented separate lists to the second meeting of the International Statistical Congress, held in Paris in 1855. D'Espine's list grouped causes according to their nature, that is, as gouty, herpetic, hematic, etc., while Farr's list was arranged under five groups: epidemic diseases, constitutional (general) diseases, local diseases arranged according to anatomical site, developmental diseases, and diseases directly resulting from violence. The president of the committee that discussed the lists stated that classification or grouping of the diseases had only secondary importance; the main point was to produce a list of morbid entities frequent enough to merit the attention of the statistician, enabling comparison of data on known morbid entities.

This Second Congress adopted a compromise list of causes of death that underwent a number of revisions but did not receive international acceptance. However, the general arrangement and structure of the list originally proposed by Farr, including the principle of classifying diseases by etiology followed by anatomic site, survives in the present classification.

The list prepared by the committee listed conditions under the following headings only:

I. Stillbirths (item 1)
II. Deaths from congenital debility, malformations or monstrosity (items 2–7)
III. Deaths from old age (item 8)
IV. Deaths from accident or violence (items 9–14)
V. Deaths from well-defined diseases (items 15–111) (The first 32 items correspond to Farr's group of epidemic diseases and d'Espine's "Acute specific" diseases.)
VI. Deaths from ill-defined diseases or described only by symptoms (items 112–138)
VII. Deaths from unknown cause (item 139)

The resolutions of this congress also recommended that each country should ask for information on causes of death from the doctor who had been attending the deceased, and that each country should take measures to ensure that all deaths were verified by doctors.

The 1855 list does not seem to have achieved much acceptance, except in the sense that its "morbid entities" figured in most lists used by countries, even if not in the same order. The subject was discussed at decreasing intervals over the next 36 years. The 1855 list was revised in 1857, the main change being the combining of classes V and VI into a heading called "Deaths from well-defined diseases" and rearrangement of the items under that heading. The items were arranged in no particular order,

it being remarked that a rigorous classification, even if established with great difficulty, would never satisfy all demands; it was "based instead on practical principles." A resolution was also passed that countries should require that causes of death be reported by doctors who should use the nomenclature items and no others—a forlorn hope, even at that time.

The congress meeting in 1860 in Paris discussed hospital statistics and adopted a complete statistical layout for classifying hospital cases, using a list of causes said to be based on the 1855 Paris list and the same as used by Farr at the General Register Office for England and Wales for many years; in fact, the Paris list corresponded more closely with that of d'Espine. The driving force in this discussion was Nightingale, who also proposed a very elaborate plan aimed at demonstrating statistically how improved sanitary conditions and better schooling reduced mortality, illness, and even criminal behavior.

The 1863 meeting of the International Statistical Congress in Berlin considered a classification for Army statistics of diseases, which had little connection with the earlier lists. In 1864 in Paris, the list of causes of death was revised according to Farr's model, with diseases organized by anatomical site; it was revised in 1874, 1880, and 1886. Nevertheless, by the end of the 1880s, most countries and cities where statistics were produced used their own lists, although the most important of them followed Farr's general pattern and listed diseases anatomically.

Bertillon classification

The 1891 ISI meeting in Vienna marked the beginning of true international acceptance of statistical lists of causes of death and sickness. Jacques Bertillon, Chief of Statistics for the City of Paris and grandson of Achille Guillard, who had instigated the 1853 decision to investigate a uniform disease classification, presented the assembly with a classification of occupations. He was asked to chair a committee that would prepare a list for causes of death at the next ISI meeting, which took place in 1893 in Chicago. Bertillon presented his report on "nomenclature of diseases (causes of death and incapacity for work, including hospital admissions)." He had been asked to produce two or three lists, of which the shorter summarized the longer, so that each administration could choose a more or less detailed list without upsetting comparisons.

Bertillon presented three lists of 44, 99, and 161 conditions with subdivisions designated A, B, C, etc. The conditions in the two longer lists, which never or rarely caused death, were printed in italics. In explaining the principles behind the structure of his classification, Bertillon remarked that Rayer in 1855 had been right to stress the importance of the individual diseases listed. Bertillon included group headings mainly for convenience and had not paid undue attention to editing them. Groupings concerning the nature of diseases tended to lose meaning over time, while individual diseases remained identifiable and ideas about them changed only slowly. Bertillon had, therefore, adopted for main headings the anatomical site rather than the nature of disease, according to Farr's plan, as had all the main lists in use. Bertillon's list included defined diseases most worthy of study by reason of their transmissible nature or their frequency of occurrence.

Bertillon's main headings were:
I.   General diseases
II.   Diseases of nervous system and sense organs
III. Diseases of circulatory system
IV.   Diseases of respiratory system
V.   Diseases of digestive system
VI.   Diseases of genitourinary system
VII. Puerperal diseases
VIII. Diseases of skin and annexes
IX.   Diseases of locomotor organs
X.   Malformations
XI.   Diseases of early infancy
XII. Diseases of old age
XIII. Effects of external causes
XIV. Ill-defined diseases

Residual categories, "other diseases of …," were provided where appropriate. The first part of General Diseases, section I, lists "epidemic diseases," i.e., acute infective diseases; some chronic infections, including tuberculosis and syphilis, appear later in the list. Both tuberculosis and syphilis have subrubrics concerning the site. Bertillon explained that he felt it was better to group all tuberculosis together and subdivide it according to site, than to distribute tuberculosis of various organs to the various anatomical headings. In several places in his discussion of his classification, he points out the advantage of listing next to each other those diseases between which the distinction was not clear, and of putting certain ill-defined conditions near their probable causes—stirrings of some of the principles followed in subsequent international classifications. Cancer was given a rubric subdivided according to site.

Bertillon stated that he had already started work on his classification in 1885 and that it had been tried out successfully since then in Paris and used in other French towns. He had commenced his work by extracting from commonly used dictionaries all of the diseases listed, allocating them to the above groups, and selecting the most important for specific rubrics. In addition, for the benefit of clerks analyzing the documents in the French towns preparing statistics, he had prepared "a sort of medical dictionary" showing to which rubric each of the diseases belonged—in effect devising the equivalent to a first

version of the Alphabetical Index, which continues to be an integral component of ICD.

Bertillon also prepared some rules or guidelines on the resolution of problems; for example, how statistical clerks should classify what is written without imputing what the doctor might have meant, and what to do when the site is not mentioned or when an operation is written as a cause of death. Another guidance dealt with how to classify cause of death when certificates mention two causes.

The three versions of Bertillon's classification received general approval, effectively marking the inception of the *International List of Causes of Death*; a small Committee on Health Statistics was set up to finalize the lists in the hope that they would be adopted by all countries.

The report of the committee chaired by Bertillon was submitted and adopted by ISI at its meeting in Chicago in 1893. Publication of this report was the origin of the *International List of Causes of Death.*

By the time of ISI's 1899 meeting, the Bertillon cause-of-death classification had been published in French, English, Spanish, and German, and Bertillon was able to report that the classification had made considerable progress; he referred to the classification at this stage as a "uniform nomenclature of causes of death." It had been adopted in the whole of North America (United States, Canada, Mexico), in several parts of South America, and in some cities in Europe. Egypt, Japan, and Algeria were said to be studying it, and most European countries were interested but did not want to change their existing lists. In all, it was a "brilliant success" for ISI.

The American Public Health Association (APHA) at its meeting in October 1897 had recommended adoption of the Bertillon classification by all registrars of vital statistics in the United States, Canada, and Mexico. An alliance of countries in the Americas using the classification was established and produced an English version. In September 1898, APHA passed a resolution that the classification be revised every 10 years, to keep up with the progress of medical science. The revision would be entrusted to an international committee, for which "strict regulations" were set out, which was to meet in Paris in 1900. APHA entreated that as many countries as possible make known their adoption of the classification to be in a position to take part in the revision and place 20th century statistics on a uniform and comparable basis. Shortly afterward, at APHA's request, Bertillon wrote to statistical administrations in Europe, which often governed individual towns, asking for their observations on the classification, whether they would adopt it for the statistics for which they were responsible, and whether their country would adopt it as a general measure. He told the 1899 ISI session that he had already received lengthy, well-researched, and interesting responses, some well-founded but needing further medical as well as statistical technical study.

The 1899 ISI session passed the following resolution (19):

The International Statistical Institute convinced of the necessity of the use in different countries of comparable nomenclatures;

Learns with pleasure of the adoption by all the statistical administrations of North America, by a part of those in South America and a part of those in Europe, of the system of nomenclature presented to it in 1893;

Strongly insists that the system of nomenclature be adopted in principle and without revision by the statistical institutions of the whole of Europe;

Approves, at least in its broad lines, the system of decennial revision proposed by the American Public Health Association in its session at Ottawa (1898); and

Enlists the statistical administrations who have not yet adopted it to do so without delay, and to contribute to the uniformity of nomenclature of causes of death.

APHA's resolutions on preparing for the revision asked countries to solicit suggestions for change from demographers, clinicians, pathologists, public health experts, and all those who use mortality statistics, stressing the importance of continuity to keep changes to an indispensable minimum. Lastly, the countries that had adopted the classification were requested to send a delegation to the revision conference. These constituted the blueprint for a revision procedure that has been followed over time.

The proposed voting system on revisions, that is, one vote per 1,000 registered deaths and a two-thirds majority for any changes, did not seem to have been necessary. The revision conferences were meticulously prepared and the delegates were presented with drafts of the revised classification in a form that already reflected a consensus. Therefore, voting was rarely necessary.

First Revision—1900 (in use 1900–1909)

Early in the history of the *International List of Causes of Death*, a revision cycle was established to keep the list abreast of medical progress. In 1899, ISI approved the proposal made by APHA for the decennial revision of the list. This provided a means of updating the classification system and meeting new needs for a disease classification. As a result of this resolution, the French government, under the auspices of the International Congress of Hygiene and

Demography, convoked the first International Conference for the Revision of the International List of Causes of Death in Paris on August 18, 1900.

Bertillon had prepared a revised draft after collating the many observations he had collected. Some reservations were expressed, notably on the headings of the main sections and on the allocation of diseases to the various sections. Bertillon explained that the headings were for convenience only and were absent in the shortest list. The delegates formally agreed to recommend to their governments adoption of the classification beginning January 1, 1901 (20), and to recommend that the French government, absent other arrangements, call the next conference in 1910.

The First Revision (ICD–1) had the same basic structure as Bertillon's original list, except that the first main heading was replaced by two subheadings, one for Epidemic Diseases and one for Other General Diseases. The list excluded stillbirths. Only two versions continued, a Detailed list and an Abridged list, the intermediate-length list having been dropped (although retained in the United States). Although the list was designed for causes of death, a parallel list for causes of sickness (morbidity) could be derived by including some additional subrubrics.

ICD–1 was translated from the original French into several other languages, alphabetical indexes were prepared, and use of ICD–1 spread quite rapidly. It was adopted even in countries that had not sent delegates to the revision conference. By 1909, Bertillon was able to report to the ISI meeting in Paris that ICD–1 was in use throughout the world, in the Americas, Australia, and Japan. He commented that Europe was more refractory and that "the countries want to be comparable with each other but above all comparable with themselves." Nevertheless, ICD–1 was in use in all eastern Europe and some other countries— Spain, France, Belgium, the Netherlands, Bulgaria, in some cities in Austria-Hungary, and in St. Petersburg and some other Russian towns. In Britain, local Sanitary Authorities were using the classification, even though the Registrar-General's offices were still using their own development of Farr's list. Bertillon was appointed director of an International Bureau of Vital Statistics to continue his work on the classification and its revision.

| 13 |

Second Revision—1909 (in use 1910–1920)

The Second Revision (ICD–2) showed for the first time "inclusion terms," that is, extra terms to be classified to the rubrics and indicating their scope. Appended to the list were Bertillon's notes on the resolution of problems in classifying causes of death and on dealing with certificates recording more than one cause.

The conference for the Second Revision, planned for 1910, was moved forward to 1909 at the request of the U.S. Census Office responsible for U.S. mortality statistics. The Census Office needed the revision available for death rates based on population data from the 1910 census. The conference was held July 1–3, 1909, in Paris under the auspices of the government of France.

As before, Bertillon had circulated revision proposals to all statistical authorities who might be interested and had meticulously prepared for the revision. By that time, a conservative estimate had the classification in use for classifying causes of death for a population of more than 212 million. It was noted that "all English-speaking and Spanish-speaking countries of the world were united in their adoption of the International List." This included all the countries on the American continent, Australia, China, Japan, and British India in Asia; Egypt, Algeria, and South Africa in Africa; and many countries of Europe.

ICD–2 represented no basic change in the structure of the list, except for the addition of a section on causes of stillbirths. It was called the *International Classification of Causes of Sickness and Causes of Death* and comprised a detailed list and an abridged list, with the causes of morbidity being designated only by letters.

The main changes were identification of many more individual diseases, especially in the General Diseases section; separate rubrics for additional anatomical sites; and rearrangement of the External Causes section to include categories for the main types of violence such as falls, cutting and piercing, crushing, etc.

Notes on causes of death that were difficult to classify and on how to deal with certificates with more than one cause were again included along the lines of the rules that Bertillon appended to his 1893 classification.

The Second Revision Conference had recognized that a special list of names of diseases would have to be prepared for each language into which the list was translated, since a direct translation of the French words was not always meaningful in other languages. Each language sometimes has alternative names for the same condition, a concept that was surprisingly difficult to communicate and continues to present problems in the present day.

The English translation of ICD–2 prepared by the U.S. Bureau of the Census commented for the first time on use of the words "nomenclature" and "classification" to describe the list. The revisions were not a true nomenclature in the sense of a complete list of conditions with a description, nor were they a classification except in the sense of statistical titles to permit comparison. For this reason, the U.S. manual was called the *International List of Causes of Death*. The English language version of ICD–2 also contained a much expanded Alphabetical Index, because a simple index was recognized to be inadequate. To prepare the Alphabetical Index, a number of nomenclatures were searched for disease names with the help of many people, including T.H.C. Stevenson, Medical Statistician of the Registrar-General's Office in London. After a special conference with Bertillon in Paris, an index covering 1,044 typewritten pages of 30 lines each was prepared. This index showed the source of the items and gave the rubric numbers of both the detailed and abridged lists. Its preparation was described as "no light task," a sentiment echoed by those who have been involved in preparing alphabetical indexes over the years.

ICD–2 met with great success. It was adopted for use beginning in 1911 by the Registrars-General of England and Wales, Scotland, and Ireland (21). Copies of the classification were distributed by the Colonial Office throughout the British Empire, where complete registration of vital events was said to be enforced. Although many countries, including the United States, had adopted the classification, it was not always being used by all jurisdictions within the respective countries.

Third Revision—1920 (in use 1921–1929)

World War I delayed the conference for the Third Revision (ICD–3) until October 11–15, 1920. Bertillon had circulated the revision proposals to more than 500 people known for their work in nosology, statistics, and public health. As usual, he prepared for the conference in minute detail with a systematic analysis of the comments received on the proposed revisions.

Many changes were made to the detailed list and new rubrics were identified, notably:

- Cerebral atheroma was separated from cerebral hemorrhage and transferred from the Diseases of the Nervous System to arteriosclerosis in the section on Diseases of the Circulatory System.

- In the section on General Diseases, provision was made for disorders of various endocrine glands, most of which had not been previously identified.

- In the Digestive Diseases section, intestinal parasitic diseases were mentioned for the first time.

- Some changes were made in the section on Childbirth; puerperal hemorrhage evidently included hemorrhage of pregnancy.

The convention signed after the conference recommended that ICD–3 be adopted by countries as of January 1, 1922, and if possible, as of January 1, 1921. Shortly after the revision conference, before he could prepare the definitive version of the Third Revision as adopted with inclusion terms, Bertillon became seriously ill. He had to hand over the work on the revision to Knud Stouman of the League of Red Cross Societies, who soon afterward took a prominent post with the newly established League of Nations. Because this resulted in some delay, countries had to prepare their 1921 statistics lists with only partial knowledge of the inclusion terms for the rubrics. The final completed version of ICD–3 was not available in French until 1923. Forty-three countries adopted this revision (22).

Fourth Revision—1929 (in use 1930–1938)

Bertillon died soon after the Third Revision Conference. At the ISI session in Brussels in 1923, Michel Huber, Director of Statistics for France, noted that Bertillon's death left a void difficult to fill, but the best memorial would be to ensure continuance of his work. Preparations soon commenced for the revision due in 1929. ISI resolved to reconstitute its Sanitary Committee, originally set up in 1893. Some medical personalities were added as members, and the augmented committee met in Paris in April 1927 to consider the next revision.

The committee reviewed the classification structure and decided that it was premature to adopt a classification giving greater emphasis to etiology. It therefore agreed to retain Farr's and Bertillon's idea of a classification with a preponderance of categories devoted to diseases by anatomical site. However, the international list already contained a number of etiological agents in the infectious diseases section. The committee recognized that it would be possible to transfer disease categories progressively to an etiological basis with the accumulation of knowledge about etiology of diseases.

The committee felt that the broad lines of the classification should be retained but suggested subdividing the General Diseases section into distinct groups. Members expressed the view that disease descriptions consisting of a noun qualified by an adjective should be classified according to the adjective (apart from "alcoholic"), i.e., giving precedence to etiology. This decision established an important principle that guided subsequent revisions. The

ISI meeting in Cairo in December 1927 adopted proposals for the revision based on these recommendations. In the meantime, the Health Section of the League of Nations had appointed a Committee of Statistical Experts which had also been concerned with the revision and communicated with governments on the matter. This may have created a certain tension during this period between ISI, in whose province the classification had resided to that point, and the newly created League of Nations section, which felt it their proper province, especially since the league's Health Section represented a more medical viewpoint.

The French government circulated ISI's proposals to governments asking for their comments and inviting delegates to the next revision conference to be held in October 1929. After an exchange of letters between the French Foreign Ministry and the Secretary General of the League of Nations, it was decided that coordination of the responses from the various governments and preparation of the final draft proposals for the Fourth Revision (ICD–4) should be undertaken by a Mixed Commission, with four members each from ISI and the League of Nations, ISI's director, and the president of the League's Health Committee attending. The Mixed Commission met in Paris in April 1929 to consider all of the observations and proposals that had been made, notably detailed comments from ISI, APHA, Austria, Great Britain, and the Netherlands. The commission then formulated draft proposals for ICD–4.

The conference for the Fourth Decennial Revision took place again in Paris, during October 16–19, 1929, with delegations from 38 countries. The conference adopted a detailed list of causes of death, 155 rubrics in all, and an abridged list of 42 rubrics (23). It reinstated Bertillon's proposal of an intermediate list of 86 rubrics, which had been dropped in the 1900 classification but had been widely seen as desirable. The detailed list, or at least the intermediate list, was recommended for use by countries. The abridged list was seen as applicable to certain uses such as tabulation of mortality data by month, population subgroups, and small geographic subdivisions.

Thirteen rubrics for causes of stillbirth, in three groups, were annexed. The main changes in ICD–4 were:

- The title for Section I was changed to Infectious and Parasitic Diseases. Separate rubrics for diseases where deaths occurred in only a few countries were deleted, with the specification that the number of deaths from the individual diseases should be shown in footnotes under this title. Parasitic diseases were transferred to Section I from other parts of the classification.

- The section on General Diseases was divided, and the following sections were created into which various diseases were transferred from other parts of the classification:

II.   Cancer and other tumors
III. Rheumatism, Diseases of Nutrition and of Endocrine Glands, and Other General Diseases
IV.   Diseases of Blood and Blood-forming Organs
V.   Chronic Poisoning

- Gangrene was moved from Diseases of the Skin into the section on Diseases of the Circulatory System.

- Section XI, Pregnancy, Childbirth and Puerperium, was completely rearranged and rationalized. Toxemia and placenta praevia were listed for the first time.

- Section XIV, Congenital Malformations, contained only one main category. Individual malformations were identified as subcategories.

- In Section XI, Diseases of Early Infancy, premature birth and injury at birth were listed separately.

- Section XVII, Violent and Accidental Deaths, was reduced to three rubrics for Suicide, Homicide and Accidents with obligatory subrubrics. A separate table was recommended for accidents according to place of accident.

E. Roesle, Chief of the Medical Statistical Service of the German Health Bureau, had in 1927 published a study of the expansion of ICD–3 that would be required in order to compile morbidity statistics. However, it was decided to deal only with causes of death in ICD–4.

The Mixed Commission recommended that a study of comparability of mortality statistics be made during the transition period by coding data for one or several years using both the old and new revisions of the classification.

The ISI session in 1929 recommended that the Mixed Commission prepare the next revision to avoid having several overlapping committees.

Fifth Revision—1938 (in use 1939–1948)

The Fifth Decennial Revision Conference was held October 3–7, 1938, in Paris with delegates from 22 countries and five international organizations in attendance. The conference decided to give weight to the practical considerations of comparability, while accepting that some changes were necessary for scientific reasons. Separate rubrics were provided, as much as possible, for the diseases that were moved from one group to another. The conference adopted a detailed list of 200 rubrics, an intermediate list of 87 causes of death, and an abridged list of 44 with an additional 14 causes of stillbirth (24).

The main changes were:

- In Section I, infectious diseases were arranged in the order of bacterial, spirochetal, filtrating viral, rickettsial, protozoal, helminthial, fungal, and other infective or parasitic diseases. Tabes dorsalis and general paralysis were transferred from Diseases of the Central Nervous System to syphilis in this section.

- In Section II, Cancer, new categories were added, including one for nonmalignant tumors and one for tumors unspecified as to malignancy.

- In Section III, avitaminoses were moved from this section to the end of the classification.

- Section IV, Nervous System, was rearranged because of the transfers of Tabes dorsalis and General Paralysis, but many numbers remained the same.

- Section XI, Diseases of pregnancy, childbirth, and the puerperium, was rearranged on the advice of a special committee but retained the same range of code numbers.

- In Section XVIII, Violent and Accidental Deaths, the rubrics for Suicide were contracted to make room for transport, machine, and mine and quarry accidents. The section assumed a structure that evolved into the present External Causes of Accident chapter.

- A total of 44 rubrics was retained by adding many optional subdivisions that would have to be used by countries wishing to retain comparability with ICD–4.

- Some occupational and nonoccupational subcategories were introduced for certain diseases of occupational origin.

The Fifth Revision (ICD–5) became a model for subsequent revisions. The conference recommended a study of comparability by the dual classification of deaths occurring in 1940 using both ICD–4 and ICD–5 to provide a bridge between the two.

Sixth Revision—1948 (in use 1949–1957)

The Sixth Revision (ICD–6) was a major revision in terms of both content and range of application. The scope of ICD–6 expanded to explicitly apply to morbidity as well as mortality; the concept of a primary cause of death for tabulation was refined and operationalized; and the legal authority of the classification was strengthened and formalized.

World events had a role in changing the organizations involved in developing ICD–6. Shortly after the Fifth

Revision Conference in 1938, World War II began and led to the demise of the League of Nations, which had played a major role along with ISI and the French government in the decennial revisions of the *International List of Causes of Death*. At the conclusion of the war, the Interim Commission of WHO, which had assumed the functions of the League of Nations on the decennial revisions of the international list, undertook the preparatory work for ICD–6.

In 1945, taking cognizance of a resolution of the Fifth Decennial Revision Conference, the U.S. Department of State constituted the U.S. Committee on Joint Causes of Death to 1) study various means of unifying the methods of selection of the main cause of death to be tabulated when two or more causes are reported on the death certificate, and 2) develop a morbidity classification. Consideration of the issues involved in a morbidity classification was particularly important as development of national morbidity statistics gained ground.

The U.S. committee included representatives from Canada and the United States, with experts from the United Kingdom and the Interim Commission of WHO serving in an advisory capacity. At the committee's first meeting December 11–13, 1945, it was noted that considerable advances had been made, particularly in developing morbidity statistics in Canada, the United Kingdom, and the United States. Each country found it necessary to devise its own morbidity classification because existing codes were impractical for the statistical classification of causes of illness.

A morbidity classification scheme proposed by the U.S. Bureau of the Budget was submitted to the committee to meet the needs of federal agencies for a disease classification. This proposal was to be considered with other existing codes, namely, the Standard Morbidity Code for Canada (25), the U.S. Public Health Service diagnostic code (26), and the British Medical Research Council morbidity classification (27).

The committee agreed that the classification to be developed would be a combined morbidity and mortality list for statistical purposes. The general arrangement of the *International List of Causes of Death* was to be followed as closely as feasible without destroying the value of the morbidity list. Some consideration was also to be given to the comparability of mortality time series. For the numbering system, one hundred 2-digit codes were proposed, with each code bearing, as much as possible, statistical meaning in terms of the rubrics covered and frequency of reporting. The 2-digit codes would be further subdivided into 3-digit classifications. For some rubrics, a 4-digit subdivision was to be considered.

Details of the combined morbidity and mortality classification were entrusted to a subcommittee of representatives from England, Canada, and the United States, which met in Washington, D.C., in the spring of 1946 to prepare a statistical classification of illness, injuries, and causes of death in accordance with the principles outlined by the U.S. Committee on Joint Causes of Death. The subcommittee also prepared a Tabular List of inclusion terms and a brief Alphabetic Index so that the classification could be subject to field trials.

The draft classification was then tested on mortality and morbidity data in Canada, England, and Wales, and in the United States. The problems encountered in these field trials were studied by the subcommittee, and necessary modifications were made. The committee as a whole gave its approval to the *Statistical Classification of Diseases, Injuries and Causes of Death* at its meeting held in Ottawa on March 10, 1947. This meeting was followed by a joint meeting of the U.S. Committee on Joint Causes of Death and the International Committee for the Preparation of ICD–6. To carry out its responsibility, the chairman of the international committee requested that the U.S. committee make available its work for review and study. Upon considering the suggested amendments to the tabular list of inclusion terms, the international committee proposed to the Interim Commission of WHO that the list of categories of the *International Statistical Classification of Diseases and Causes of Death* be submitted to governments with the recommendation that the classification be adopted as the basis for the Sixth Decennial Revision of the International Lists of Causes of Death.

The Sixth Decennial Conference for the Revision of the International Lists of Diseases and Causes of Death was convened by WHO and the French government in Paris during April 26–30, 1948. The task of the conference was to consider adopting the statistical classification as developed in two sessions of the Expert Committee on Health Statistics of WHO. The proposed classification represented an expansion of the previous international lists to provide specific categories for nonfatal diseases and injuries. The classification contained approximately 800 categories when injuries were classified according to the nature of injury, that is, physiological consequence (e.g., fracture of the femur) and 765 when they were classified according to the external cause of injury (e.g., a fall).

The numbering system employed in ICD–6 was a departure from the combined 3-digit number and an alphabetical subdivision used in the earlier revisions. The numbering system provided greater flexibility and made possible the introduction of new categories in later revisions without greatly upsetting the basic numbering of other categories. It also lent itself to statistical operations involving large volumes of records.

The titles of the 17 main sections of ICD–6 did not differ greatly from the 18 groupings of ICD–5. The sections "Senility" and "Ill-defined Conditions" were combined into a single section, and Section V, "Chronic Poisoning and Intoxication," of ICD–5 was eliminated. In its place, a new main grouping "Mental, Psychoneurotic and Personality Disorders" was introduced. Lastly, provisions were made for the dual classification (external cause of injury and nature of injury) of the section on "Accidents, Poisonings and Violence." The external cause classification was the primary one to be used for cause-of-death statistics.

Also introduced in ICD–6 was a recommended format for recording causes of death designed to elicit from the physician, among reported causes, the underlying or initiating cause that would be used for tabulating official statistics on cause of death. Further, coding rules for selecting, and in some cases modifying, the underlying cause of death were clearly articulated with examples.

The Sixth Revision Conference approved the proposed classification and recommended publication of the *Manual of the International Classification of Diseases, Injuries and Causes of Death* in two volumes: Volume I would contain, in addition to the Introduction, the List of Categories and a Tabular List of Inclusion Terms, a section on medical certification, coding rules for mortality classification, and special lists for tabulation. Volume II would contain a comprehensive alphabetic list of diagnoses and conditions. For the first time, English-speaking countries would be using the same classification manual, which would be a further aid for comparability of international statistics.

Because of the effectiveness of the U.S. Committee on Joint Causes of Death in producing the groundwork for ICD–6, in the form of a combined morbidity and mortality classification and in unifying the method for selecting the underlying cause of death, the U.S. delegation proposed to the conference that national committees on vital and health statistics be established in all countries to study issues and problems for the development and production of vital and health statistics. The conference passed a resolution recommending the formation of such national committees in member countries. The First World Health Assembly adopted the Sixth Revision of the *Statistical Classification of Diseases, Injuries, and Causes of Death* on July 24, 1948, to go into effect on January 1, 1950 (28).

Seventh Revision—1955 (in use 1958–1967)

A significant development in 1951 was the establishment of the first WHO Center for Classification of Diseases at the General Register Office of England and Wales in London. The center was to serve as a clearinghouse for problems in the use of ICD and for questions on application of the rules for coding the underlying cause of death, and to assist the WHO Secretariat in the development of ICD in a setting where data were available for testing revision proposals.

Because ICD–6 represented a major change from previous revisions, it was expected that the Seventh Revision (ICD–7) would be limited to minor adjustments, giving countries time to implement the changes, and to adopt the classification for morbidity. Hospitals, especially in the United States, found ICD–6 useful for indexing medical records. In addition, WHO's Expert Committee on Health Statistics recommended that decennial revisions of the classification be held in the years ending in "5" so that the revised classification could be applied to mortality statistics at the beginning of years ending in "8." This would make it possible for countries to accumulate sufficient experience in using the new classification before population figures became available from decennial national censuses, usually held in years ending in "0" or "1," to serve as a base for mortality studies. This proposed change in the revision cycle would cut short the time available for preparatory revision work, providing another reason to limit ICD–7 to essential changes and amendment of errors and inconsistencies.

Revision proposals were prepared by the WHO Advisory Group on Classification of Diseases and circulated to countries for comment. The suggestions received were reviewed by the Expert Committee on Health Statistics, which adopted suggested modifications consistent with the limited scope of the proposed revision. The International Conference for the Seventh Revision of the International Statistical Classification of Diseases and Causes of Death was held in Paris on February 21–26, 1955, and the classification was formally adopted (29,30). The Revision Conference did not believe it was the right time to formulate specific rules for the classification of morbidity data and agreed with the Expert Committee on Health Statistics that more information was required on the different types of morbidity statistics for which coding rules were needed.

Aware of the experience of a number of countries in expanding ICD for use as a diagnostic index for hospital histories, and recognizing that ICD was suitable for such use, the conference recommended that the revised manual of the classification include a note explaining the principles that should be followed in expanding ICD for use as a diagnostic cross-index.

Eighth Revision—1965
(in use 1968–1978)

At the time of ICD–7, it was anticipated that a major change would be made at the Eighth Revision (ICD–8). In the United States, preparatory work started in 1958 when the National Committee on Vital and Health Statistics appointed subcommittees to study and propose revisions of various ICD sections. Early in the 1960s, several other national administrations and regional organizations initiated studies of different chapters of the classification.

Development of ICD–8 was influenced by the adaptations of ICD–7 to meet the needs of hospitals in several countries, notably Israel, Sweden, and the United States, for diagnostic indexing of clinical records. In addition, the Pan American Health Organization (PAHO), the regional organization for WHO in the Americas, published a Spanish translation of the U.S. Adaptation of ICD–7 for use in hospitals in Latin American countries.

WHO's Expert Committee on Health Statistics was entrusted with the task of studying the various revision proposals submitted for international consideration and recommending a classification of diseases that would serve as the basis for ICD–8. This task was made particularly difficult by the unprecedented number of suggestions for modifications. Many of the major revision proposals involved different axes of classification, and it was not always possible to arrive at a compromise solution.

In reviewing the various purposes for which ICD was being used, the Subcommittee on Classification of Diseases of the Expert Committee on Health Statistics reiterated the view that the basic function of ICD is to classify data on causes of morbidity and mortality for statistical purposes. However, the subcommittee also recommended that this not prejudice its use for other needs such as indexing diagnostic data for storage and retrieval in hospitals. The subcommittee considered in detail the revision proposals that were received from countries. Preliminary revision proposals for these and other sections were prepared and submitted to national administrations for study and comment.

The final preparatory meeting of the WHO Expert Committee on Health Statistics was held in November 1964. The committee reviewed the different classification sections, made decisions on major issues, and gave guidance on other problems to be dealt with by the WHO Secretariat.

The International Conference for the Eighth Revision of the ICD was held July 6–12, 1965, in Geneva (31). Major revisions were made in several ICD sections, namely, infective and parasitic diseases, mental disorders, diseases of the circulatory system, congenital malformations, diseases and conditions occurring in the perinatal period, and the nature of injury and external causes of accidents, poisoning, and violence.

The changes in the classification of infective and parasitic diseases reflected mainly current knowledge of viral diseases with a consequent expansion of the classification relating to these diseases. Extensive 4-digit subdivisions were provided to show the various clinical manifestations of zoonotic bacterial diseases such as plague, tularemia, and anthrax, and of the spirochetal and mycotic diseases. An important change in this revision was the transfer of diarrheal diseases to this section. A similar proposal made for transferring influenza and pneumonia was not adopted.

The classification of diseases of the circulatory system, once the center of a stormy discussion, was settled without controversy. A significant change was the transfer of the cerebrovascular diseases to this section from the Diseases of the Nervous System and Sense Organs. Another major change was the provision of 4-digit subdivisions to show the association between hypertension and cerebrovascular diseases and ischemic heart disease.

The former section on "Certain Diseases of Early Infancy" was merged with the "Supplemental Classification on Causes of Stillbirth" to form the new section "Certain Causes of Perinatal Morbidity and Mortality." This change gives recognition to the continuum between conditions in the fetal and early neonatal periods.

The classification of the nature of injury was expanded to provide greater detail on adverse effects of drugs and other substances. The classification of external cause of injury (E-code) gave more emphasis to the circumstances surrounding accidental falls and fires. It also identified the agent, or the more common hazards, in the Western world. The E-code also provided for classification of those events where the circumstances surrounding the death (i.e., accident, suicide, or homicide) could not be determined after a medicolegal investigation.

At the request of WHO, NCHS in the United States undertook preparation of the Alphabetical Index to ICD–8. This task was accomplished as a collaborative effort involving personnel from NCHS; WHO; the WHO Center for the Classification of Diseases in London; health departments of Georgia, Michigan, and Virginia; National Institutes of Health; Office of the Surgeon General; Department of the Army; and American Hospital Association (AHA).

ICD–8 was approved by the International Conference for the Eighth Revision of the ICD held in Geneva during July 6–12, 1965 (31), and went into effect on January 1, 1968, for the compilation of national morbidity and mortality statistics (32).

Ninth Revision—1975
(in use 1979–1994)

WHO called a meeting of the Study Group on Classification of Diseases in October 1969 to advise on the requirements of a program for the Ninth Revision of the ICD (ICD–9). Included in the study group were the heads of the WHO Collaborating Centers for the Classification of Diseases that had been established in London, Paris, Moscow, and Caracas (WHO centers were subsequently established in Washington, D.C.; Sao Paolo; and Beijing. Center heads met between study group and Expert Committee meetings to develop revision proposals from the suggestions received for modification of ICD).

The study group recommended that ICD–9 be a minor revision, as it followed the fairly extensive changes in ICD–8. It also recommended that the mortality orientation of the classification and assumptions of etiology be discontinued and that multiple conditions be coded separately rather than in combination categories in the classification. It was again recommended that ICD–9 serve the needs of hospitals for indexing diagnoses for the storage and retrieval of clinical records for case studies. This would require a single-axis classification and provision of a classification of items such as elective operative and treatment procedures, complications of medical and surgical procedures, symptomatology, and other causes of hospital admission not covered by diagnoses of physical and psychiatric illnesses.

In preparing for ICD–9, the WHO Secretariat sought the views of consultants, international organizations of medical specialists, heads of WHO Collaborating Centers for the Classification of Diseases, and various program units within WHO. The third meeting of the study group considered revision proposals received from all of these sources, as well as member states.

The first major issue of ICD–9 concerned the scope of the revision. Numerous suggestions were received in response to the invitation for comments, particularly from medical specialists interested in using ICD for retrieval of medical records for clinical studies, which required specific and detailed information about diseases in their specialty. Their revision proposals exceeded the initial decision to keep ICD–9 one of nominal change.

The second major issue was how to accommodate the needs of medical care programs. It was agreed that for purposes of medical treatment, the condition, not the etiologic agent, was of concern. Because ICD is basically a classification whose major axis of classification is etiology, a proposal was made to classify certain conditions twice—once according to etiology and again according to manifestation. These two codes were to be distinguished by a dagger and an asterisk, thus producing what were, in effect, two overlapping classifications. The etiology code was specified to be used for mortality tabulations.

The International Conference for the Ninth Revision of the ICD, held in Geneva during September 30–October 6, 1975 (33), adopted ICD–9 (34). The general arrangement of ICD–9 was much the same as in ICD–8, although it provided greater detail. ICD–9 comprised 909 disease categories and 192 rubrics for external causes of injuries compared with 858 disease categories and 182 E-codes (external cause of injury classification) in ICD–8.

ICD–9 incorporated the following innovations:

- Optional 5th-digit codes were provided in certain places, for example, for the mode of diagnosis in tuberculosis, method of delivery in Chapter XI, anatomical sites in musculoskeletal disorders, and place of accident in the E-code.

- An independent 4-digit coding system was provided for the classification of the histological type of neoplasms, prefixed by the letter M for morphology and followed by a 5th-digit behavior code for optional use.

- The role of the E-code was changed from an alternative classification to a supplemental classification. The prefix N, for nature of injury, was dropped, and the classification of nature of injury became part of the main classification. The E-code was specified to be used, where relevant, in conjunction with codes from any part of the classification. However, for mortality statistics, the E-code was still to be used in preference to the nature of injury (Chapter XVII) in presenting the underlying cause of death when only one axis of classification was employed.

- Dual classification of certain diagnostic statements was implemented according to manifestation and etiology. Etiology codes were indicated by a dagger and considered primary. Manifestations of certain diseases were marked by an asterisk, a secondary code, to be used in the planning and evaluation of medical care.

- Categories in the Mental Disorders chapter included a narrative description of the contents to facilitate use because no standardized international terminology existed for mental disorders. This additional text indicated the intended content of the rubrics and is similar to that which appeared in the *Manual of the American Psychiatric Association* (35).

The Ninth Revision Conference also recommended that a provisional classification of therapeutic, diagnostic, and prophylactic procedures in medicine—including surgical, radiological, laboratory, and other medical procedures—be published as a supplement to but not an integral part of ICD–9. It also recommended that an Impairments and Handicaps Classification be published for trial purposes as a supplement to but not an integral part of the Ninth Revision (36).

Three ICD adaptations designed for the use of specialists were called to the conference's attention: oncology, dentistry, and ophthalmology. The oncology adaptation (ICD-O) included three axes denoting topography, morphology, and behavior of the tumors (37,38). The 4-digit topography code was based on the list of anatomical sites of the malignant neoplasms in Chapter II of the Ninth Revision. Another 4-digit code for histological type would be added, followed by a 1-digit code for behavior of the neoplasm. The ICD-O was designed as an alternative to ICD–9 for use by cancer centers, which required additional details on tumors. ICD-O codes are convertible to conventional ICD codes. The history of ICD-O, including its origin, as well as comparability between ICD-O and ICD codes, are discussed by Percy (39).

The adaptation for dentistry and stomatology was produced by the responsible WHO unit, and that for ophthalmology by the American Academy of Ophthalmology and Otolaryngology (40). All of the diseases and conditions of interest to specialists in these areas had been pulled together from various parts of ICD. A 5th-digit code was also provided for additional detail.

Tenth Revision—1989 (in use 1995 to present)

Preparatory work for ICD–6 through ICD–8 had been largely undertaken by an Expert Committee on Classification of Diseases appointed by WHO. Because of the increasing complexity of ICD–9, the heads of the Collaborating Centers on Classification of Diseases assisted the WHO Secretariat in preparing revision proposals for consideration by the Expert Committee. The role of the Collaborating Centers increased further in preparing the Tenth Revision (ICD–10).

The Expert Committee met in 1984 and 1987 to provide policy guidance and "to make decisions on the direction of the work and the form of the final proposals." The preparatory work was undertaken with a view toward making extensive modifications in ICD's structure "to serve a wide variety of needs for mortality and health care data." Experiments with various biaxial structures demonstrated that the traditional organization of ICD could not be improved. Therefore, attention was turned toward achieving a better balance in the various sections or

chapters of the classification and providing room for future expansion without disrupting the existing code structure. The usual extensive consultation process took place involving the same types of organizations and medical specialties as in ICD–9. Draft proposals were twice circulated to member countries before the final draft was presented to the revision conference.

The International Conference for the Tenth Revision of the ICD met in Geneva during September 26–October 2, 1989 (41). The conference recommended that the proposed revised chapters, with their 3-character categories and 4-character subcategories, and the Short Tabulation Lists for Morbidity and Mortality constitute the Tenth Revision of *International Statistical Classification of Diseases and Related Health Problems*. The World Health Assembly adopted ICD–10 to go into force on January 1, 1993. However, implementation was delayed until after publication of the Alphabetic Index in 1994, the Tabular List having been published in 1992 (17). ICD–10 was translated into the official languages of the United Nations, and into other languages by countries using ICD.

ICD–10 differed from ICD–9 in a number of important respects. Among the major changes were introduction of an alphanumeric coding scheme (a letter followed by three numbers at the 4-character level) to replace the numeric scheme used in ICD–9. This permitted more than double the size of the coding frame compared with the previous revision. Of the 26 available letters, 25 were used. The letter U was left vacant for future additions and changes, and for possible interim classification of problem cases arising between decennial revisions. Additionally in ICD–10, the concept of a "Family of Classifications" was developed further and a continuous updating process was introduced (see following section).

Chapter order in ICD–10 was much the same as in ICD–9 and, in accordance with the new alphanumeric scheme, the chapters are given codes prefixed by letters of the alphabet. The shifting of disease categories between chapters as well as the creation of new sections brought the total number of chapters to 21. Major changes were made in:

V.   Mental and Behavioral Disorders
XIX.   Injury, Poisoning and Certain Other External Causes
XX.   External Causes of Morbidity and Mortality

The dual classification scheme for etiology and manifestations introduced in ICD–9 was modified and extended to 82 homogeneous 3-digit categories for optional use. With this change, diagnostic statements containing information about both a generalized underlying disease process and a manifestation or complication relating to a particular organ or site could now be double-coded so that retrieval or tabulation can be made by axis, etiology, or manifestation. In addition, exclusion notes at the beginning of each chapter were expanded to explain the relative hierarchy of chapters, and to make clear that the special group chapters that bring together, for example, all neoplasms and all trauma, have priority of assignment over the organ or system chapters. Among the special group chapters, those on "Pregnancy, Childbirth, and the Puerperium" and on "Certain Conditions Originating in the Perinatal Period" have priority over the others.

At the beginning of each chapter, an overview is given to the block of 3-digit categories and, when relevant, to the asterisk categories. This addition clarifies the chapter structure and facilitates use of asterisk categories.

ICD–10 is much more detailed than ICD–9, continuing the process of increasing detail particularly to meet the needs of morbidity. ICD–10 has expanded to about 8,000 categories compared with nearly 5,000 in ICD–9, showing more information for many types and sites of disease; in a few cases, less detail is shown.

In ICD–10, some category titles have been changed and regrouped. Examples of title changes include the ICD–9 title Chronic obstructive pulmonary diseases and allied conditions, which became Chronic lower respiratory diseases. Suicide became intentional self-harm, and Homicide become Assault. Notable regroupings include some cerebrovascular disorders, specifically transient cerebral ischemic attacks, which was moved from Diseases of the circulatory system in ICD–9 to Diseases of the nervous system. Septic shock, classified in ICD–9 as Shock without mention of trauma in the chapter Symptoms, signs, and ill-defined conditions was reclassified to Unspecified septicemia. Respiratory failure was moved from Symptoms, signs, and ill-defined conditions to Diseases of the respiratory system. Transport accidents were regrouped by the characteristics of the injured person rather than by the type of vehicle involved in the accident.

Continuous updating

Recognition of the need for a different approach was announced at the Tenth Revision Conference with recommendations for more frequent than decennial updating of ICD in response to largely nonstatistical needs: "… WHO should endorse the concept of an updating process between revisions and give consideration as to how an effective updating mechanism could be put in place" (17). The World Health Assembly approved of having WHO develop a mechanism for considering and implementing ICD–10 modifications in the interim period between revisions.

Subsequently, WHO and the heads of Collaborating Centers agreed to implement an annual updating process

on a pilot basis for three years, effective with the 1997 annual meeting of the heads of Centers (42). At this meeting, a working group, building on a proposal of the Secretariat, proposed that two groups comprise the updating mechanism: an "Update Reference Committee," later renamed the Update and Revision Committee (URC), composed of members drawn from clinicians, nosologists, and users of statistics and a balance of mortality and morbidity expertise. The URC would finalize recommendations for submission to the meetings of center heads. URC would be supported on mortality matters by a Mortality Reference Group (MRG) of expert members—MRG would make decisions on the application and interpretation of ICD and propose changes to the classification and mortality coding rules to URC. On the morbidity side, proposals to URC would come from the Collaborating Centers, to whom national offices and other users could refer problems. In 2006, more reference groups, including a Morbidity Reference Group, were established.

A number of process issues such as dissemination of updates have taken longer to resolve (43). For example, as of 2003, WHO had not disseminated many of the changes in either electronic form on the WHO/ICD website or in printed format, but the changes had been incorporated into the ACME software used by a number of countries for producing annual mortality files. More recently, WHO has been publishing changes from the continuous updating process in an amended edition of ICD–10 issued periodically, while electronic details on updates are available from: http://www.who.int/classifications/icd/en/ and more specifically from: http://www.who.int/classifications/icd/icd10updates/en/index.html. An evaluation of the updating arrangements was planned after 3 years' experience, with center heads taking the evaluation's results into account before deciding to start the process for the Eleventh Revision (42).

CHAPTER 4

Classifying Diseases for Primary Mortality Tabulations and Problems of Joint Causes of Death

The final prerequisite for being able to produce statistics on cause of death is to have a way to identify a single cause of death. The term "cause of death" has been a simple and convenient term to describe the disease or other morbid condition responsible for death. However, in practice, the term has many meanings in both a technical as well as colloquial context. To some medical certifiers, the cause of death may be the disease under treatment or a complication of the disease; to others, the cause of death is the terminal disease or the mode of dying. Frequently, symptoms and ill-defined descriptors are reported as causes of death. Many years were required to achieve consensus on the meaning of the term for statistical purposes, and to devise a data collection instrument—the international medical certificate—that could be depended on to elicit a cause of death that is reasonably reliable and comparable among certifiers, across geographic areas, and over time. Even so, variability continues to exist in the diagnostic acumen of certifiers, in styles of medical certification, and in the care with which diagnostic information is reported on death certificates.

The medical certificate section—usually on a death certificate and sometimes a "death notification form"—used to collect information from the physician who certifies the cause-of-death information on the diseases and other conditions involved in a death, follows a standard international format prescribed in the current ICD version and called the International Form of Medical Certificate of Death (17). The cause-of-death information reported on the form is subsequently coded and classified using the current revision of ICD, a process that uses a set of international coding rules also specified in the current ICD revision. Thus, the basic tools for compiling cause-of-death statistics are: 1) the medical certificate form, 2) rules for coding causes of death, and 3) the classification of diseases and causes of death. These tools have been reviewed and revised at each decennial conference for the revision of ICD, and, effective with ICD–10, are being reviewed annually as part of the continuous ICD updating process.

This chapter discusses the concept of the cause of death, the nature of its ambiguities, and how these were reflected from the beginning of mortality statistics in both data collection and processing. The chapter traces these historical developments as they were reflected in the development and refinement of the medical certificate of death and the coding rules for selecting and modifying the underlying cause of death, which is used to tabulate and analyze "primary," or single-cause, mortality statistics. Also discussed is the application of automation in the United States in the 1970s to process cause of death, a development that standardized coding and resulted in the routine production of multiple cause-of-death statistics in the United States and other countries that have implemented the U.S. system. A final section of this chapter discusses approaches to collecting cause-of-death information for developing countries.

Concept of cause of death

"These mumps is different. It's a new kind, Miss Mary Jane said."

"How's it a new kind?"

"Because it's mixed up with other things."

"What other things?"

"Well, measles, and whooping-cough, and erysiplas, and consumption, and yaller janders, and brain-fever, and I don't know what all."

...

"Well, what in the nation do they call it the MUMPS for?"

"Why, because it IS the mumps. That's what it starts with."

"Well, ther' ain't no sense in it. A body might stump his toe, and take pison, and fall down the well, and break his neck, and bust his brains out, and somebody come along and ask what killed him, and some numskull up and say, 'Why, he stumped his TOE.' Would ther' be any sense in that? NO. And ther' ain't no sense in THIS, nuther."

—Huckleberry Finn, Susan, and the hare-lip, Chapter XXVIII, *The Adventures of Huckleberry Finn,* 1885

This fictional conversation in a Mark Twain classic captures the essence of the problem of medically certifying and classifying causes of death (44). A collection of concurrent diseases—mumps, measles, whooping cough, and others—illustrates the kind of problem faced by a medical certifier completing a medical certificate of causes of death, that is, what and how causes of death should be reported. And how is the underlying cause of death determined after neck and skull fractures result from falling down a well upon ingesting a poison? Clearly, attribution of death to "stumped his toe" as the underlying cause is reaching too far back in the sequence of events.

A key problem of medical certification of death is ascertaining the single condition of most relevance for statistical and analytical uses. Farr recognized this as a problem in compiling mortality statistics (45): "It must be stated, moreover, that the causes of death assigned are often inadequate and frequently erroneous. A person is dead. What was the cause of his death is the question addressed to the medical attendant. He has all the information to guide him in his answer that he employed during his life in the treatment; but that may be insufficient. Some few years ago 'dropsy' would have been returned, and was accepted by the medical profession as a disease, a cause of death. It is still used rightly in some cases. But many cases are traced back further; the dropsy is found 1) to be associated with albuminous urine, and affections of the kidney, such as Bright's disease; or, 2) it is the result of retarded circulation from organic disease of the heart; or 3) it is ascites, an effusion into the peritoneal sac from obstructed circulation ... or 6) it is the consequence of scarlet fever; 7) it is anaemic; or 8) it comes on suddenly with fever; or 9) it is general and associated with scurvy. Now after the first step is made in defining the seat and source of the 'dropsy' we have got at one link of the chain of causes. The dropsy or scurvy, or anaemia, may be traced to famine, or to insufficiency of some elements of diet; that cause is primary. Then the scarlet fever is the cause of dropsy; but what is the cause of the first disease? How was the dead child infected? Ascites, the cirrhosis of the liver, may be traced to alcoholism as its primary cause; or the heart disease may be derived from rheumatic fever. And the rheumatic fever may be the result of exposure to malaria of a specific kind. Now in many cases the primary cause can, but in many cases it cannot be discovered. Yet to be able to prevent death, the primary cause is of first importance, as it sets the rest in motion."

The conceptual complexity of determining cause of death was articulated more recently by the eminent biostatistician Raymond Pearl, who noted (46), "Philosophically considered, a true determination of the 'cause of death' is in a great many cases, indeed probably the majority of all cases, an extraordinarily difficult matter. The difficulty arises from many different circumstances. Some

illustrations will perhaps make the point clear. A woman has cancer of the breast, is operated on in hope of curing this disease, develops postoperative pneumonia and dies. Now if the woman had not had the cancer and therefore not been operated on for its relief, this train of circumstances would not have gotten underway. This way of looking at the matter plainly suggests that the cancer was fundamentally the cause of death. But, on the other hand, if she had not been operated on, even though she still had the cancer, she would not have died when she did, but at some later time. This view rather tends to make the operation the cause of death, at least at the particular time and place at which it occurred. Again, suppose she had been operated on, and had not developed the postoperative pneumonia, then she might have been permanently cured of the cancer (some are) and lived to a ripe old age. This view of the case truly makes pneumonia the cause of death. Which of these things—cancer, operation or pneumonia—is to be charged as the primary cause of death plainly depends upon the point of view, or, put in another way, upon what definitions or rules are set up as to what is called the cause of death."

The aforementioned examples by Twain, Farr, and Pearl demonstrate long-standing recognition of the conceptual difficulty of defining a meaningful cause of death. Was it to be the cause that initiated the sequence of events that led to death, or was it to be the terminal condition? Or was it to be the condition that was greatest in severity, or longest in duration? Not only what was it, but for what purpose? Would the cause of death most useful for legal purposes be the same as the cause most meaningful for public health purposes?

How to capture a statistically and legally meaningful cause of death evolved gradually over a period of five decades, through trial and error and experimentation with different formats in different countries. Part of the problem was that of jointly reported causes recognized by Bertillon, who formulated rules and guidelines to help select a single cause under these circumstances. However, a comprehensive solution required that the death certificate itself be designed to reduce ambiguity and to elicit diagnostic information that corresponded to a sought-after concept of cause of death. This was gradually achieved through successive revisions by changes in the recommended death certificate format, culminating in ICD–6 of the international certificate, which has remained largely unchanged through ICD–10.

Medical certificate of cause of death

At the beginning of the 20th century, considerable variability existed in the format of the medical certificate adopted by various countries, but the report of the Health

Committee of the League of Nations suggests that some countries were using similar certificates that nonetheless varied in wording. According to the Health Committee, in countries like France, Germany, and the Netherlands, only the cause of death was asked for without any suggestion to the medical certifier that the reporting of more than one cause was inappropriate. No instructions were given as to what the certifier should report as the cause of death. In many countries, the medical certificate forms used suggested that, in appropriate cases, more than one cause should be specified. However, this suggestion was stated in different ways, which was certain to result in different kinds of response.

Some forms called for 1) the principal cause and 2) contributory causes, but no information was required as to the relationship between the reported causes, except that one was more important than the rest. In most countries, the forms asked for the mutual relationship between the reported causes, but this was not always done in the same way.

The Second Revision of ICD as adopted by the United States mentions that the certificate used in England and Wales and the medical certificate recommended by APHA were practically identical. Both asked for statements of causal relationship, but the issue was obscured by alternatively calling them causes of importance. In England and Wales, the terms "primary" and "secondary" were defined as referring to a causal relationship, but the medical certificate was so worded that the second cause could not be secondary but contributory. Therefore, it was impossible to tell, however carefully and well the form was filled out, whether the relationship between the reported causes was that of causation or of importance. The U.S. standard death certificate at that time presented the same kind of problem. The medical certificate called for 1) the cause of death and 2) contributory (secondary) cause (Figure 1). The main heading of "the cause of death" gave no indication as to whether it was the primary or principal cause of death. Cause of death was defined as the "primary cause of death" in the instructions to medical certifiers on the back of the death certificate. The two relationships of causation and importance also were confused by the addition of the parenthetical term "secondary" to the contributory cause. In the 1910 and 1918 (Figures 2 and 3) revisions of the medical certificate, the following note was appended: "State the Disease Causing Death, or, in Death from Violent Causes, state 1) MEANS OF INJURY, and 2) whether ACCIDENTAL, SUICIDAL, or HOMICIDAL."

In 1925, Stevenson submitted for the Health Committee's consideration a medical certificate form to bring about greater uniformity in the forms being used by different countries. This form differed from the earlier formats in two respects. First, the part of the certificate that had been

Figure 1. U.S. Medical Certification Section, 1900

Figure 2. U.S. Medical Certification Section, 1910

called the "Cause of Death" or "Primary Cause of Death" was changed to "Principal Cause of Death." Second, subdivisions were created under the Principal Cause of Death, lines (a), (b), (c), and (d), for reporting the sequence of events leading to death.

The medical certificate form recommended by the Health Committee of the League of Nations at the Fourth Revision Conference was adopted by England and Wales in 1927

Figure 3. U.S. Medical Certification Section, 1918

MEDICAL CERTIFICATE OF DEATH

16 DATE OF DEATH (month, day, and year)   19

17   I HEREBY CERTIFY, That I attended deceased from

..................., 19......, to ...., 19......

that I last saw h----- alive on ----------------------, 19......

and that death occurred, on the date stated above, at .... m.
The CAUSE OF DEATH* was as follows:

------------------------(duration) .... yrs. .... mos. .... ds.

CONTRIBUTORY---------------------------------------
(SECONDARY)
-----------------------(duration) ..... yrs. ..... mos. ..... ds.

18 Where was disease contracted
    if not at place of death?-------------------------------

Did an operation precede death? .... Date of ....

Was there an autopsy?------------------------------------

What test confirmed diagnosis? ----------------------------

   (Signed)... M. D.

   , 19   (Address)

* State the DISEASE CAUSING DEATH, or in deaths from VIOLENT CAUSES, state
(1) MEANS and NATURE of INJURY, and (2) whether ACCIDENTAL, SUICIDAL, or
HOMICIDAL. (See reverse side for additional space.)

Figure 4. U.S. Medical Certification Section, 1930

MEDICAL CERTIFICATE OF DEATH

21. DATE OF DEATH (month, day, and year)   193

22.   I HEREBY CERTIFY, That I attended deceased from

...................................., 193 , to ...., 193

I last saw h ----- alive on ----------------------------, 193 ; death is said

to have occurred on the date stated above, at ---------- m.
The principal cause of death and related causes of importance were as follows:
                           Date of onset

--- ----------

--- ----------

--- ----------

--- ----------

Other contributory causes of importance:

--- ----------

--- ----------

--- ----------

Name of operation ------------------------ Date of------------

What test confirmed diagnosis?------------------ Was there an autopsy?--------

23. If death was due to external causes (violence), fill in also the following:

Accident, suicide, or homicide?------------ Date of injury ----------- 193

Where did injury occur? --------------------------------------
             (Specify city or town, county, and State):
Specify whether injury occurred in industry, in home, or in public place:

Manner of injury --------------------------------------

Nature of injury ---------------------------------------

24. Was disease or injury in any way related to occupation of deceased?----------------

If so, specify ---

(Signed) ---

(Address) --

and by Canada in 1935. In the United States, the wording of the medical certificate was changed in 1930 from "Cause of death" to "Principal cause of death and related causes of importance" (Figure 4), but no provision was made for reporting the sequence of events leading to death in accordance with the international recommendation. The Health Committee made a clear semantic difference between the primary and principal causes of death. Although this is probably a valid distinction, many countries did not appreciate the difference in meaning between the two terms.

Starting with the 1930 revision of the U.S. standard death certificate, specific questions on the circumstances surrounding injuries were made part of the medical certificate form. This made possible the compilation of better statistics on the external causes of injury.

Addition of "related causes of importance" in the United States was presumably in lieu of lines (a), (b), (c), and (d), which were omitted in the 1930 U.S. standard death certificate. This omission was rectified a decade later, and the 1939 U.S. standard death certificate called for reporting the sequence of events leading to death (Figure 5). However, the heading "principal cause of death" as recommended by the Health Committee was not adopted.

Figure 5. U.S. Medical Certification Section, 1939

MEDICAL CERTIFICATION

20. Date of death: Month ------------ day------------

    year ------------ hour ---------- minute -----------

21. I hereby certify that I attended the deceased from----------

------------------, 19---, to ----------------, 19---:

that I last saw h------ alive on ------------------ 19---:

and that death occurred on the date and hour stated above.   *Duration*

Immediate cause of death ------------------------------

Due to --

Due to --

Other conditions ----------------------------------   PHYSICIAN
    (Include pregnancy within 3 months of death)

Major findings: Underline
   Of operations ------------------------------ the cause to
                                  which death
                                  should be
   Of autopsy------------------------------- charged sta-
                                  tistically.

22. If death was due to external causes, fill in the following:

(a) Accident, suicide, or homicide (specify) -----------------

(b) Date of occurrence----------------------------------

(c) Where did injury occur? ----------------------------------
                     (City or town)   (County)   (State)

(d) Did injury occur in or about home, on farm, in industrial place, in public

    place? ---
                              (Specify type of place)
    While at work? ---------- (e) Means of injury -----------

23. Signature -------------------------- (M. D. or other)---

Address-------------------------------- Date signed -----

The medical certificate adopted in the United States in 1939 omitted reference to the principal and contributory causes of death. It starts with the immediate cause of death, followed by the antecedent causes. Instead of referring to contributory causes, the item simply calls for "other conditions."

A number of other innovations were made in the 1939 revision of the U.S. medical certificate. Because confidence was lacking that American medical certifiers would fill out such a form correctly, a note was added to the U.S. certificate instructing the physician to "underline the cause to which the death should be charged statistically." A study by Joseph DePorte later showed that in a large proportion of cases, the medical certifiers in New York were ignoring this instruction on underlining (47). DePorte concluded that it was impractical to obtain from physicians their opinion about the underlying cause of death by means such as underlining; the instruction to underline was deleted at the next decennial revision of the U.S. standard death certificate.

Another innovation was the parenthetical note attached to other (contributory) conditions to "include pregnancy within 3 months of death." This was added to flag possible maternal deaths which might otherwise be missed in the statement of causes of death. Yet another addition was a provision for recording the major findings of operations.

The Fifth Decennial Revision Conference adopted the medical certificate form recommended by the Health Committee. Instead of calling for the "primary cause of death and the contributory causes of death," the recommended medical certificate asked for the "principal and the independent contributory cause of death" (not causally related to the principal). The first item to be reported under the principal cause of death was the immediate cause of death, followed by antecedent morbid conditions, if any, that gave rise to the immediate cause of death. The last stated cause in this sequence of events was to be the underlying cause of death. A note was appended to this format that states, "In most cases, it would suffice to state the principal cause, reserving statement of contributory causes for instances where the deceased succumbed to a combination of maladies none of which would necessarily have been fatal by itself. In such cases, the certifier's judgment alone could afford guidance as to the cause to be selected as principal, i.e., the cause chiefly contributing to the death and under which the death should be tabulated."

The change in wording of the medical certificate from cause of death to principal cause of death represented a basic change in concept from causation of death to the importance of the cause of death. However, it is not clear whether the intent was to switch from causation to importance or to induce the medical certifiers to report only the important causes of death. Vital statistics offices were having difficulties with reports of signs and symptoms, ill-defined diseases, and trivial conditions as the cause of death. The change in wording to principal cause of death may well have been an effort to encourage certifiers to report the more important disease entities.

The Sixth Revision Conference recommended adopting the form proposed at the Fifth Revision Conference except that the main heading "principal cause of death" was deleted, as was line (d). The first part was formally labeled Part I and the contributory causes Part II (Figure 6).

For the first time, adoption of the international medical certificate of causes of death by the signatory nations of WHO became obligatory, in accordance with the provisions of Regulations No. 1 of ICD–6.

Figure 6. U.S. Medical Certification Section, 1949

MEDICAL CERTIFICATION

18. CAUSE OF DEATH
Enter only one cause per line for (a), (b), and (c)

** This does not mean the mode of dying, such as heart failure, asthenia, etc. It means the disease, injury, or complication which caused death.*

I. DISEASE OR CONDITION DIRECTLY LEADING TO DEATH* (a) ____

ANTECEDENT CAUSES
Morbid conditions, if any, giving rise to the above cause (a) stating the underlying cause last.
DUE TO (b) ____
DUE TO (c) ____

II. OTHER SIGNIFICANT CONDITIONS
Conditions contributing to the death but not related to the disease or condition causing death.

INTERVAL BETWEEN ONSET AND DEATH

19a. DATE OF OPERATION | 19b. MAJOR FINDINGS OF OPERATION | 20. AUTOPSY? YES ☐ NO ☐

21a. ACCIDENT SUICIDE HOMICIDE (Specify) | 21b. PLACE OF INJURY (e.g., in or about home, farm, factory, street, office bldg., etc.) | 21c. (CITY, TOWN, OR TOWNSHIP) (COUNTY) (STATE)

21d. TIME OF INJURY (Month) (Day) (Year) (Hour) m. | 21e. INJURY OCCURRED WHILE AT WORK ☐ NOT WHILE AT WORK ☐ | 21f. HOW DID INJURY OCCUR?

22. *I hereby certify that I attended the deceased from ____, 19__, to ____, 19__, that I last saw the deceased alive on ____, 19__, and that death occurred at ____m., from the causes and on the date stated above.*

23a. SIGNATURE (Degree or title) | 23b. ADDRESS | 23c. DATE SIGNED

The international medical certificate remained unchanged from ICD–6 to ICD–9, as did the main features of the medical portion of the U.S. Standard Certificate of Death (Figures 7–9). At the Tenth Revision Conference, another line (d) was added to Part I of the medical certificate, in line with earlier guidelines from WHO and following

adoption of a fourth line in the 1989 revision of the U.S. Standard Certificate of Death (48).

The 1948 revision of the U.S. Standard Certificate of Death and the medical format subsequently in use in the United States basically follow the internationally recommended form. However, items related to operations, autopsy, or

Figure 7. U.S. Medical Certification Section, 1956

Figure 8. U.S. Medical Certification Section, 1968

Figure 9. U.S. Medical Certification Section, 1978

violence that have been on versions of the U.S. form over time are not included in the international medical certificate. The U.S. standard death certificates of 1989 and 2003 (Figures 10 and 11) further added detailed instructions to guide the medical certifier in completing cause of death, including examples of properly completed certifications (48).

The death certificate developed for 2003 is largely similar to that of 1989, except for the inclusion of a pregnancy item as recommended in ICD, more detailed instructions, a tobacco use item, and minor modifications in other items. Additional information is available from the NCHS website: http://www.cdc.gov/nchs/nvss/vital_certificate_revisions.htm.

Figure 10. U.S. Medical Certification Section, 1989

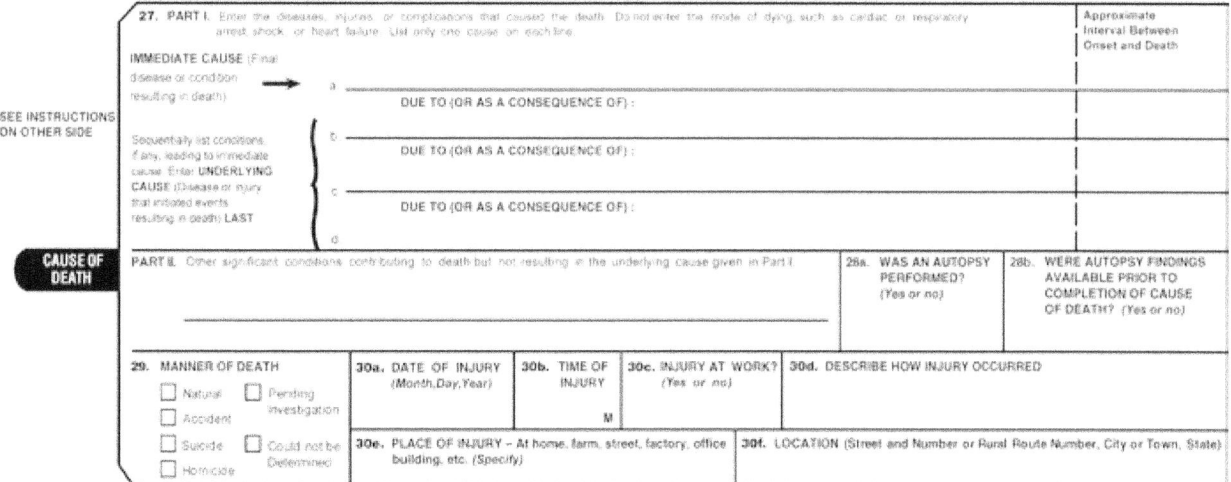

| 29 |

Figure 11. U.S. Medical Certification Section, 2003

Coding rules for selection and modification of underlying cause of death

A major and long-standing problem in compiling official mortality statistics results from physicians reporting two or more causes of death on the death certificate. It is, according to ICD–1 (20), "one of the most annoying and difficult subjects, for a wholly satisfactory solution, that occurs in the practical compilation of mortality statistics. It is very common for the physician to report two or more causes of death in connection with a given case, which causes may perhaps sustain a certain relation to each other, as primary or secondary, direct or indirect, chief or determining, and consecutive or contributory, or be wholly unrelated so far as the statement received at the compiling office may indicate. For most statistical purposes, no matter how many contributory causes may be assigned by the physician, the choice of causes of death is restricted to a single cause."

Billings made the same point in ICD–1 (20), "All systems of mortality statistics are compiled on the principle that the number of cases of death and causes of death must be the same. So long as this is the case, it is practically impossible to give a full view of the causes of death. In other words, binomial or polynomial returns as originally made by the physician [i.e., more than a single cause of death—authors' note] must be forced into tables constructed on a monomial basis, and it sometimes happens that the fuller and more explicit the original statement of cause of death the greater may be the difficulty that will be experienced in the assignment to a single title of the classification."

The problem of joint causes was explicitly recognized by Bertillon, who devised an initial set of guidelines or rules to guide coders in selecting the single cause of death for tabulation. Application of these rules, which were refined over time, varied widely among countries until WHO mandated the use of ICD rules under WHO Regulations No. 1. Tracing the rationale for these rules is central to understanding their development.

Selecting the underlying cause of death

At the First Revision Conference on the International List of Causes of Death in 1900, Bertillon prepared, as a guide to medical officers responsible for determining the cause of death, a commentary on the most frequent complications of selected diseases and the complications that should not be taken into account (49). The commentary was appended to the French version of the 1900 revision of the *International List of Causes of Death*. Bertillon also formulated general rules for use when two or more causes of death are reported jointly:

"Rule 1. If one of the two diseases is an immediate and frequent complication of the other, the death should be classified under the heading of the primary disease. Examples:

- Infantile diarrhea and convulsions, classify as diarrhea.

- Measles and bronchopneumonia, classify as measles.

- Scarlet fever and diphtheria, classify as scarlet fever.

- Scarlet fever and nephritis, classify as scarlet fever.

"Rule 2. If it is not absolutely certain that one of the diseases is an immediate result of the other, we must see if there is a very great difference in the gravity of the two, and classify the death under the heading of the more dangerous. Examples:

- Cancer and bronchopneumonia, classify as cancer.

- Pulmonary tuberculosis and puerperal septicemia, classify as tuberculosis.

- Icteris gravis and pericarditis, classify as icteris gravis.

"Rule 3. When among the two causes of death there is a transmittable disease, it is preferable to assign the death to it, for statistics of infectious diseases are particularly interesting to the sanitarian, and it is important that they shall be as complete as possible.

"Rule 4. If a disease whose evolution is rapid is given in connection with another whose evolution is slow, it is preferable to charge the death to the first. Again, if a death is simultaneously attributed to an external violence, it is usually proper to assign it to the latter.

"Rule 5. Finally, if none of the preceding rules is applicable, the diagnosis most characteristic of the case should be selected."

Bertillon gave the highest priority to acts of violence. He also emphasized the importance of infectious diseases, which were of special interest to sanitarians of that period. The rest of the rules were designed to get at the primary disease rather than complications or the mode of dying. Finally, a provision was made to attribute the death to the most appropriate category.

These rules were not formally adopted by the International Revision Conference, but they served as guides for the various national vital statistics offices. The United States and a number of other countries put into practice various modifications of Bertillon's proposed rules.

Manual of joint causes

In many instances, Bertillon's selection rules were simple to apply. However, many cases occurred where the rules proved inadequate and decisions had to be made as to which of the causes should be selected for primary mortality tabulations. These decisions were recorded, enabling consistency in the cause-of-death assignment each time that the same combination of diseases or conditions was jointly reported. In 1914, the U.S. Bureau of the Census, which was then responsible for the compilation of national vital statistics, published an *Index of Joint Causes of Death* based on all joint-cause decisions, numbering in the thousands, that had been made up to that time (50).

The *Index of Joint Causes of Death* was printed in proof to indicate the provisional character of some of the decisions and to enlist the constructive criticism of workers in the field of practical statistics before preparing a more definitive index or method of treatment. The index comprised a series of tables that showed which disease or condition had priority when jointly reported. When more than two diseases were jointly reported and the tables did not show which disease had a clear priority over the others, the coder referred to a separate manual for instructions on tie-breaking. These comprehensive instruction manuals for cause-of-death coders were issued annually.

In 1925, a revision of the *Index of Joint Causes of Death* was issued as the *Manual of Joint Causes of Death* (51). The 1925 ICD revision states that, "As the treatment of joint causes of death has never been adequately treated by anybody, the second *Manual of Joint Causes of Death* is published as a temporary guide for those who are groping for help in making their assignments, rather than an authoritative manual."

In 1939, the joint-cause manual was incorporated into the U.S. volume of the *International List of Causes of Death* (52,24). The 1939 manual continued to call attention to the tentative nature of the joint-cause selection rules—even after 40 years of use of this important procedure by an official agency.

Although various countries agreed to use the *International List of Causes of Death* and Bertillon's rules for selecting the primary cause of death, international uniformity was not obtained. Repeated efforts were made over many years to secure uniformity, but each country continued to make modifications to suit its special needs.

The Fourth Revision Conference requested the U.S. government to undertake a study of joint causes of death. The results showed great variations in death rates by cause for different countries, arising from the lack of uniformity in applying joint-cause rules.

No further decision was taken on the matter of joint-cause rules at the Fifth Revision Conference held in 1938, but the conference did propose for international adoption a medical certificate form that had been developed by England and Wales. In this certificate, the medical certifier was to pinpoint the underlying cause of death by the manner in which the causes of death are reported. When this medical certificate form was first adopted in the United States in 1939, the intention was to tabulate the physician's statement of the underlying cause of death. However, few believed American physicians would do any better with the new certificate than with the old. Consequently, use of the old joint-cause coding procedure continued from 1940 to 1949. Because of the uncertainty that medical certifiers were making any distinction between the entry for the cause of death and the contributory cause, the joint-cause rules were applied to all information reported on the medical certificate. This practice gave undue weight to contributory causes.

Just prior to ICD–6, the U.S. National Office of Vital Statistics faced the issue of the joint-cause coding procedure. Despite its imperfections, the joint-cause manual had served its purpose over the years. The systematic nature of the selection process and the consistency of coding were important factors in favor of its retention. On the other hand, a change was needed if full advantage was to be taken of the international form of medical certificate and the new classification procedures. A study was therefore conducted in which the same batch of death certificates was coded using: 1) the U.S. joint-cause selection procedure then in effect, 2) the same as in 1) but applied only to information reported in Part I of the medical certificate, and 3) the general rule and the modification rules as proposed for international adoption.

The study showed considerable difference between methods 1 and 3, and relatively little difference between methods 2 and 3. Furthermore, there was greater consistency between coders when using Method 2 compared with Method 3. On the basis of overall merit, the procedure applying the joint-cause rules to information reported only in Part I appeared to be the method of choice. Despite this finding, the decision was made to abandon the joint-cause manual that had been in use in the United States for 50 years and to adopt the proposed international rules, because it would be difficult to justify pursuit of an educational program for improving death certificate information if the physician's statement of causes of death (i.e., the underlying cause) was not taken into account in the classification of causes of death.

The joint-cause rules of Bertillon and the subsequent revisions had come under criticism because they did not take into consideration the opinions of the medical certifiers. The great value claimed for the international

| 31 |

medical certificate and the international rules for selecting the underlying cause of death was that the opinion of the medical certifier would be accepted as the underlying cause of death. In actual practice, this was only partially true. The statement of the underlying cause is accepted when the medical certificate is completed properly. If not, the certifier's opinion is substituted by an appropriate but arbitrary rule in order to obtain consistency in statistical tabulation and to minimize the vagaries in reporting or the omission of required medical information. This is not necessarily a bad practice—in fact, it more often than not results in what appears to be a more sensible assignment of cause of death.

Cause-of-death coding rules in Sixth Revision

The concept of the underlying cause of death and the rules for its selection were adopted at the Sixth Decennial Conference for the Revision of the International Statistical Classification of Diseases and Causes of Death in 1948. They were similar in application and principle to Bertillon's rules proposed in 1900—both were designed to get at the cause of death for single-cause tabulations. However, under WHO Regulations No. 1 issued as part of ICD–6, all of the WHO signatory nations were obliged to adopt the classification, the medical certificate of cause of death, the coding rules for selecting the underlying cause of death, tabulation lists, age groupings, etc. Unless a signatory nation of WHO enters a specific reservation, the country is bound by WHO regulations, which have the force equivalent to any international treaty or covenant. For the first time, adoption of an international procedure for coding causes of death became obligatory, thus making possible the production of internationally comparable statistics on causes of death.

Rules were formulated for selecting the underlying cause of death from the new design of the medical certificate form and were included in the WHO manual of classification. In principle, the underlying cause to be selected should be the condition recorded on the lowest line of the medical certificate. The coding rules were designed to give precedence to what the medical certifier had indicated as the underlying cause, unless 1) there were clear indications he or she had not understood the way in which the certificate was intended to be completed, or 2) the classification provided for some modification of the underlying cause to be made as a better way for presenting the death in statistical tables. That better way might involve giving preference to one jointly reported condition over another, or combining two individual diagnostic terms into a single term as listed in the classification. An example of case 2 would be a case where "essential hypertension" was recorded as the underlying cause with

an organic consequence on the line above; ICD had for some time allowed for subclassification of hypertension according to various organic consequences, and from a statistical viewpoint, showing the subclassification rather than including such a case simply under "essential hypertension" is more satisfactory.

Coding the underlying cause of death could be conceived of as a two-step process: First, the underlying cause is selected using coding rules to determine the etiological plausibility of the reported causal sequence. Second, the selected underlying cause is modified using rules that take into account considerations a) and b). In most cases, the underlying cause should be the condition reported by the certifying physician on the lowest-used line of Part I. But in some cases, the final underlying cause would differ from that reported by the physician. A study by Green using a sample of U.S. death certificates showed that the tabulated underlying cause of death agreed with the first condition reported by the physician on the lowest-used line of Part I of the death certificate about 80 percent of the time (53).

Coders were provided with selection and modification rules that came into play when certain situations arose. When a medical certificate with an impossible situation of events occurred, the only really satisfactory solution was to query the medical certifier, but this often was not possible. The selection rules were arbitrary and, in the spirit of making the best of a bad job, were designed to ensure that similar certifications were treated in the same way in all places and in all countries using them. The logic of the rules was that if the medical certifier had not understood the way in which the certificate worked, it is likely that the first thing he or she wrote or a sequence leading from it would have been uppermost in his mind as the cause of death, even if the sequence had something unconnected appended at the end. Another rule allowed coders to pick up an obvious underlying cause from Part II (e.g., primary cancer no longer present at the time of death, when the death was due to secondary cancers, or pneumonia in Part I resulting from a chronic condition reported in Part II of the death certificate).

The international rules for selecting the underlying cause of death posed a new and difficult problem for coders who needed to take cognizance of the improbable relationship between diseases and other morbid conditions sometimes reported in Part I of the medical certificate. The new coding procedures necessitated retraining nosology coders, in both the U.S. national office and state offices of vital statistics.

In the United States, a training deck was prepared to illustrate each rule in the new procedure. Training courses were organized in various regions of the country to which a coder-trainer from each state was invited. A publication titled *Nosology Guidelines* was inaugurated. Each issue discussed coding principles and some aspect of the coding procedure. Included were 10 coding problems with the question, "How Would You Code This?" followed by the answers to the problems. In case of disagreement, the state coders were invited to comment on the answers, or to request further explanation in case there were questions.

Coding rules after Sixth Revision

Cause-of-death coding rules have remained generally similar from ICD–7 to ICD–10, although some changes have been made with consequences for comparability of mortality statistics between revisions. For example, some changes were made at ICD–8 to clarify intent. ICD–9 introduced some changes, including a new rule allowing a therapeutic misadventure rather than the condition being treated to be selected as the underlying cause when it was apparent that a treatment error was responsible for the death (but not when something had simply gone wrong or the patient had reacted abnormally).

ICD–10 introduced some further clarification and changes to the selection and modification rules (54). Among these changes were consolidation of two coding rules, namely, those involving senility and ill-defined conditions; and the dropping of two rules, one regarding pneumonia, influenza, and maternal conditions, and the other for errors and accidents in medical care. The greatest impact on statistical data in ICD–10 was a change in the direct sequel rule that extended it to a much broader range of conditions. Changes were made in the selection of the primary site of cancer, and, subsequent to the official issuance of ICD–10, important changes were made in the rules on senility and ill-defined conditions, and in the instructions on improbable sequences. Changes made subsequent to ICD–10 were approved through the continuous updating process implemented by WHO beginning in 1996 (42,54,55).

Automating cause-of-death coding

Around 1970, initial steps were taken by the United States to automate cause-of-death coding, prompted by the advent and diffusion of high-speed automated computing equipment. Several reasons motivated the attempt to apply computer technology to mortality coding: 1) It was believed that the resulting coding would be more consistent and accurate than manual coding, which often reflected intercoder variability in practice and interpretation of reported diagnoses; 2) it was believed that production costs might be reduced because of simplified training and data entry; and 3) it was hoped that a by-product of automated underlying-cause coding would be the routine production of "multiple causes of death," that is, all the conditions reported by the certifying physician, not just the single underlying cause of death (56).

The present U.S. automated system for coding cause of death has four components, the first of which is the automated coding of medical entities, or ACME. Data entry requires that the coder key all of the diagnostic terms that the physician reported using a specified format and explicit coding procedures. The records then are processed automatically using ICD selection and modification rules to select the underlying cause of death in the same way that a manual coder would. The ACME component proved to be highly efficient and effective, with a capability of automatically processing more than 99 percent of the records. The small percentage of records that could not be processed automatically were manually coded, many of these being deliberate "rejects" such as maternal deaths in which careful scrutiny of individual records was desired.

ACME was used to process U.S. death records beginning with deaths occurring in 1968. In the 1980s, the ACME program was adopted by a number of countries in Western Europe, and it continues to be adopted by an increasing number of countries throughout the world. Other automated systems were developed concurrently by France, Sweden, and other countries; subsequently they, too, adopted ACME (57,58).

A second component of the U.S. system was developed and implemented shortly after ACME to produce multiple-cause data (59). Called TRANSAX for "translation of axes," the program produces up to 20 conditions per record plus the underlying cause of death, in two formats: 1) "Entity Axis" information, which represents ICD codes corresponding to all the conditions as coded into the ACME program, with line and placement on the line of each diagnostic entity encoded into the statistical record; and 2) "Record Axis" information, in which ICD codes have been subjected to the selected modification rules, and redundant codes eliminated. Record Axis codes generally are arranged on the statistical unit record in ascending ICD order. As a consequence, the order of the conditions on the death certificate is lost in Record Axis format. In the United States, multiple-cause data are available on an annual basis beginning with the 1968 data year through the present.

In implementing the automated coding systems ACME and TRANSAX in the United States, a major concern was related to costs. Although the automated system produced more consistent, reliable, and accurate coded data, the costs of the automated system were not less than that of the manual system it had replaced. Specifically, the costs of training, data entry, system maintenance, and system modification (resulting from ICD revisions and interim coding changes) exceeded those of manual underlying-cause coding. Efforts were therefore directed to developing data-entry components of the automated system that could result in reduced costs for training and data entry. By the early 1990s, two programs had been developed—the Mortality Medical Indexing, Classification, and Retrieval program known as MICAR and a subsequent refinement called SuperMICAR.

MICAR was developed in the 1980s to simplify ACME and TRANSAX data entry. MICAR was an intermediate step; it required that coders learn new, and simplified, procedures for data entry that nevertheless allowed for using a simplified or "sanitized" diagnostic vocabulary, or, alternatively, special index numbers called entity reference numbers (ERNs). MICAR was composed of two parts: an extensive dictionary of ERNs and corresponding medical terms to which terms were continuously added as they were encountered on death certificates; and the coding conventions used by NCHS for multiple-cause data entry, as spelled out in the NCHS coding manual (60).

A major advantage of MICAR for data retrieval and analysis was that each diagnostic term on the death certificate was given a unique ERN compared with ICD codes, which in many instances are summary categories that lose diagnostic detail reported on the death certificate. With MICAR, information as reported by the certifying physician could essentially be reconstructed, which cannot be done using ICD codes.

MICAR was followed in 1993 by SuperMICAR, which was the first successful program in the United States to accept for data entry "natural language," that is, the diagnostic terms exactly as reported by the physician, which subsequently could be fully processed through the sequential application of MICAR, ACME, and TRANSAX. While SuperMICAR is specific to Americanized English, variants have been developed in several other languages (56).

By the beginning of the new millennium, automated coding systems for cause of death had realized their promise of improving consistency both within and among countries using ICD for mortality classification. On the downside, the automated systems, like other complex computer algorithms, are very costly to revise when changes are required, as when ICD is revised either in a sweeping change as with the introduction of a new revision, or even on an incremental basis as a result of the new continuous-updating process. Moreover, to ensure international comparability, all countries must use the same version of ACME software. The International Collaborative Effort on Automating Mortality Statistics is playing a key role in coordinating implementation and maintenance of automated mortality coding systems among countries.

One issue confronting WHO and the international community is development of tools like SuperMICAR for languages other than English. A general solution to this problem could greatly expand international dissemination

of automated systems. For instance, IRIS is a language-independent coding system based on NCHS's system that is currently in development (61).

Automated coding systems promise to further standardize mortality data throughout the world and have the potential of making routinely available both multiple-cause data and a higher level of diagnostic detail than previously available using just ICD categories.

Cause-of-death statistics for developing countries

All of the foregoing history and discussion of causes of death relate to the production of statistics based on medical certification of causes of death. Many developing countries that could benefit greatly from statistics on causes of death lack such data because a large population does not receive medical attention. Only relatively few deaths are certified by qualified medical practitioners. The resulting statistics on causes of death are a mixture of diagnostic data with a preponderance of vague and ill-defined descriptors of causes of death. Such data cannot be meaningfully used because it is not possible to relate deaths with and without medical attention to their respective populations at risk.

Biraud was perhaps the first to propose, in 1956, a method for collecting cause-of-death information by lay personnel (62). In this system, a lay person would be trained to record symptoms and complaints which, if classified by a simple but appropriate method, could be interpreted by an epidemiologist with knowledge of the country, its lore, and pathology in such a way as to prove useful for practical action by health authorities.

In 1971, WHO held a meeting of a group to discuss the problem of using ICD for lay reporting of morbidity and mortality in developing countries. This group recommended a classification and methods of recording signs, symptoms, and complaints. In 1973, WHO convened another meeting to assess the value of lay reporting, especially with respect to information on maternal and perinatal deaths.

In 1976, the Ninth Revision Conference discussed the suitability of ICD for classifying lay reports on causes of illness and causes of death (33). The conference recommended that WHO assist countries in developing methods of using lay and paramedical personnel to collect morbidity and mortality data.

That same year, a working group convened by the WHO Regional Office for South-East Asia drew up a detailed list of symptoms recognizable by primary health personnel throughout the world. From this detailed list, two shorter lists were derived, one for causes of death and the other for reasons for contact with health services. Field trials on the use of these lists were conducted, and the results became the basis for revising the lists. WHO published these lists as an example of the lay reporting system for adaptation to other circumstances (63).

Other regional meetings on lay reporting have taken place. WHO and the United Nations Environment Program held a joint meeting in Nairobi on lay reporting of health information. In the following year, the two organizations conducted a similar meeting for French-speaking African countries in Dakar, Senegal. In 1992, WHO and UNICEF convened a meeting on lay reporting in Geneva. In 1993, the London School of Hygiene and Tropical Medicine held a workshop on adult verbal autopsy (the current terminology for lay reporting, a catchy title that unfortunately suggests the objectivity of a pathological observation that it does not possess).

In the method of lay reporting proposed by Biraud, three significant parameters may be noted: age at death, accidents and other violent deaths, and broad symptoms, anatomical site, and duration of complaints. Age at death in itself can be of considerable health significance, and he suggested broad "physiological" age groups: suckling, youths, adults, and old people. Reporting violent deaths does not require medical knowledge for diagnosis, so the circumstances of deaths involving accidents and other violence may be readily recorded by a lay person. Biraud made provisions for recording other symptoms to identify certain febrile diseases.

To Biraud's parameters may be added one other significant fact: In developing countries, one-half or more of all deaths occur among children aged under 5 years. Most of these deaths will probably be from common childhood diseases that should be recognizable by many mothers. Provisions should therefore be made for reporting these diseases in the local vernacular. Because a number of endemic and epidemic diseases affecting the local population also are familiar to the general citizenry, an attempt should be made to identify these diseases in terms of the local jargon. In other words, every effort should be made to elicit information on the common diseases that might be readily recognized by the lay population.

Symptoms and complaints should also be collected and used to derive what might be called a "reasonable" diagnosis, an approach studied by Lukovic and Ivancovic of the Stampar School of Public Health in Zagreb, Yugoslavia (64). In their approach, a special interview form devised to collect data on symptoms and complaints was administered by civil registrars at the time of death registration. The same form was also used by nurses who reinterviewed the informant at home. Quantitatively, the field nurses elicited slightly more information than did the registrars. On the other hand, the nurses missed more

causes. The procedure was well received by the registrars who felt that this additional activity added significance to their work.

The elicited data were evaluated independently by two physicians who attempted to make some kind of diagnosis. The physicians used a table of equivalents, that is, a table that showed combinations of symptoms and complaints that were equated to a diagnostic category.

Comparisons were made between the diagnoses made by the two physicians as well as between the two data sources. A comparison also was made with the information reported on the medical certification of causes of death. The symptoms review by the physicians produced diagnostic categories that agreed with those on the medical certificates in about 75 percent of the cases. This is not a particularly high proportion, but if the diagnostic data for three-quarters of the deaths without medical attention could be improved by this means, the gain seems substantial and worthwhile.

Chandramohan et al. (65) reviewed 35 published studies of lay reporting, including mortality classification, design of questionnaires, interviewers, respondents, recall periods, procedures for deriving a diagnosis, and recording single compared with multiple causes of death. Also discussed were issues about validation of results. The review concluded that available information from these studies "is inadequate to draw firm conclusion on preferred methodological approaches to verbal autopsies for adult deaths. Before these tools are used more widely for adult deaths, further research is required to compare alternative methods and to evaluate the validity of the tool in a range of settings."

It is apparent that more field studies are needed before a universally applicable method can be made available. Each country will need to tailor a procedure to suit its situation if a lay reporting system is to be established. Another important consideration concerns the completeness of registration of deaths: A lay reporting system, no matter how good, will be of marginal use in a country where registration is highly incomplete. In these countries, the development of a lay reporting system must await the improvement of death registration. Countries also need to consider issues related to investment and direction of efforts to produce statistics on cause of death. Another report describes more recent WHO efforts related to verbal autopsies (66).

| 35 |

CHAPTER 5

Multiple Cause-of-death Statistics

As described in the previous chapter, a by-product of the tools designed to elicit an underlying cause of death is multiple causes of death. Multiple causes and statistics based on multiple causes have been referenced only in a limited way in ICD revisions to date. Yet multiple cause-of-death statistics provide a useful supplement to the underlying cause statistics already described by considering all of the diagnostic information on the death certificate, thereby providing a more comprehensive picture of cause of death. This chapter describes multiple-cause statistics, their strengths and weaknesses, their availability, some considerations in their use, and several illustrations of their use. Concluding sections discuss tabulation guidelines and the use of multiple-cause information for nonstatistical purposes.

Multiple-cause data in the United States

The limitations of underlying mortality statistics have long been recognized. As previously mentioned in ICD–1, Billings commented on losing information when statistics were based on a single cause reported on death certificates (20). In ICD–2, Pikler, in his discussion of the Budapest system of mortality statistics in 1909, "has very forcefully directed attention to the importance of the study of contributory causes of death that usually are lost in compilation, but the full statement of such causes would be difficult, especially for related tables and a detailed classification in a report dealing with a large number of returns" (21).

These commentaries were made at a time when the medical certificates simply asked for the "cause of death" and sometimes the "contributory causes of death." Since then, several revisions of the medical certificate form have been made. The international death certificate recommended following ICD–5 is designed specifically to elicit from the physician the single cause of death that initiated the sequence of morbid conditions resulting in death; however, a properly completed medical certificate will include not only the underlying cause but also the causal chain that led to death, as well as other conditions

that contributed to death but were not in the causal chain. All of these reported conditions are called the "multiple causes of death" and have the potential of providing a fairly comprehensive description of the constellation of conditions that led to death. Because of these revisions and the changing pattern of mortality from infectious to chronic diseases, an increase has occurred in the amount of diagnostic information reported on death certificates that is not reflected in official mortality statistics based on the underlying, or primary, causes of death. The obvious solution to the limitations of underlying cause statistics was to code and tabulate all of the diagnostic information reported on the death certificate.

Coding multiple-cause information is challenging because it requires deciding *a priori* how best to process all diagnostic information on the death certificate in a manner suitable for multiple-cause tabulation. In the United States, the first set of multiple-cause tabulations was for data year 1917, when one cause in addition to the underlying cause of death was coded and tabulated. Similar tabulations were made in 1925, 1936, and 1940. For data year 1955, a 50 percent sample of death certificates was coded up to a maximum of five reported entries of causes of death in the medical certificate. The multiple-cause tabulations prepared from 1917 through 1955 were not edited to eliminate duplicate counts of diseases and conditions. Nor were counts of diseases and conditions made for each death. Therefore, the resulting data are of limited use for analytical purposes.

The set of coding procedures used in the United States beginning with 1968 data is the TRANSAX automated coding program. As discussed in the last chapter, TRANSAX produces multiple-cause information in two forms, as Entity Axis codes and as Record Axis codes. Entity Axis codes represent each coded condition on the death certificate by its position in terms of the line and position on the line of the death certificate. In contrast, Record Axis codes are translations of Entity Axis codes using selected modification rules (67,68). Since the 1968 data year, NCHS has routinely produced a unit record electronic database of both multiple and underlying causes for each death in the United States, along with limited tabulations to be used principally as control totals for data users, but with some analytic applications. In addition, the data are available annually from http://www.cdc.gov/nchs/data_access/Vitalstatsonline.htm and have recently been made available from http://wonder.cdc.gov. For additional information, see the NCHS website: http://www.cdc.gov/nchs/nvss/mortality_public_use_data.htm.

Generally, Record Axis data are recommended for multiple-cause analysis and Entity Axis data for studying styles of medical certification. Entity Axis data are also used in some analytic studies, because they provide conditions prior to linkage of relevant conditions as dictated by modification rules, and therefore, in some cases, provide more detail.

Limitations of multiple-cause statistics

A basic limitation of multiple cause-of-death statistics is their sensitivity to changes in death certificate format and to the reporting practices of physicians. The international medical certificate of death was specifically designed to guide the medical certifier to report a single condition that initiated the chain of morbid events that led to death, not to obtain multiple-cause data. Consequently, multiple-cause data must be viewed as a useful by-product of the medical certification process, not as one of its goals.

Nor is the international medical form designed to obtain disease prevalence data, that is, information on all serious morbid conditions at the time of death, only those conditions that contributed to death either directly as part of a causal chain (as reported in Part I of the international form) or indirectly (Part II).

That multiple-cause data are not indicators of disease prevalence can be illustrated with mortality data on Diabetes mellitus. In 1993, a total of 64,751 deaths were attributed to Diabetes mellitus as an underlying cause. Over three times as many deaths, a total of 202,322, had a report of diabetes on the death certificate (69). Yet the prevalence of diabetes for decedents in 1993 was an estimated 411,040, based on results of the 1993 National Mortality Followback Survey (70). In other words, for only about half of the deaths for persons with diabetes was this disease reported as a multiple cause (underlying or nonunderlying cause) on the death certificate; for only 15.8 percent of decedents who had diabetes in their lifetime was diabetes selected as the underlying cause of death.

Multiple-cause data are far more sensitive than underlying cause data to the reporting practices of the certifying physician. In underlying cause statistics, the report of a single underlying cause by the physician would be adequate for tabulation purposes even if that cause, in

reality, operated through a number of intermediate but unreported conditions. The same certification would be highly incomplete for multiple-cause use, however, because it fails to communicate not only the important conditions in the causal chain but also any other significant conditions that may have contributed to the death.

Had the death certificate been designed to obtain all significant medical conditions prevalent at the time of death, the certificate probably would look very different from the international form in use today. Instead of asking for the causal sequence that led to death and other significant factors contributing to death, the certificate might ask that the certifier report all significant morbid conditions present at death, possibly by severity, duration, or relative importance. Because the purpose of the international form is not to collect multiple-cause data, the form does not request this information.

As in any kind of statistics, the completeness and accuracy with which the information is reported can also affect the counts. For example, diseases to which social stigma are attached and episodes such as therapeutic misadventures are less likely to be completely reported.

Considerations in using multiple-cause data

In tabulating and analyzing multiple-cause data, a number of decisions must be made at the outset regarding "counting." Will the subject of the counts be the total number of medical conditions reported, given that for any individual more than one condition is likely to be reported on the death certificate? Or will the subject of the counts be the number of decedents for whom a medical condition was reported regardless of whether it was selected as the underlying cause? In the former approach, traditional methods of demographic analysis cannot be used because individuals may be counted more than once, and therefore the traditional measures of risk (i.e., death rates) cannot be calculated; in the latter approach, rates can be developed because individuals are being counted, not conditions.

The basic difference between traditional underlying cause tabulations and multiple-cause tabulations in the United States from 1917 through 1955 is that underlying cause counts represent an unduplicated count of deaths by cause of death. In contrast, multiple-cause counts released prior to 1968 were counts of conditions. Thus, prior to 1968, multiple-cause tabulations and analyses were conducted using condition-counts rather than person-counts, because the files were so structured. However, from 1968 forward, the data user can make a choice regarding which approach to use with multiple-cause data and tabulate the data as either condition-counts or person-based counts. The user of multiple-cause data must also choose which tabulation lists to use. NCHS produces a number of hierarchical tabulation lists; the list chosen has consequences for multiple-cause analysis.

In addition, the analyst must make choices regarding how to handle uninformative medical information included in the multiple-cause file, in particular, modes of dying such as cardiac arrest which do not constitute meaningful diagnostic information.

The following discussion covers the considerations of condition-counts compared with person-counts, the selection of an appropriate tabulation list, and the suppression of nonmeaningful terms such as modes of dying.

Condition-counts and person-counts

To tabulate all of the information on the medical certificate for causes of death is to duplicate counts of diseases and conditions. It is, therefore, necessary to remove duplication of counts of the reported diagnostic information for each death or event, thereby making it possible, for example, to relate these events to a defined population for the computation of death rates, and to more effectively use these statistics to search for associations among conditions that are reported concurrently. Circumstances occur in which condition-counts are more appropriate than person-counts, or vice versa.

Person-based counts are more appropriate in developing multiple-cause death rates. Although underlying cause tabulations have been criticized because they do not comprehensively describe the diseases and conditions involved in the death process, they possess an important attribute—they serve as measures of the risk of dying from various causes of death. Multiple-cause data can be presented in the same manner, that is, as counts of persons with various diseases and conditions. This was proposed by Dorn and Moriyama as a means of overcoming the shortcomings of underlying cause tabulations by providing a complete count of diseases in the population of deaths (71). Multiple-cause death rates based on counts of persons or deaths can be an approximate measure of the probability of dying with note of a specific disease or combination of diseases. Nevertheless, the analyst and data user should keep in mind that the death certificate is not designed to obtain prevalence information and that consequently the probabilities are likely underestimated.

In a global count of persons with a report of a specific disease, a person or decedent may be counted more than once. For example, the medical certificate for a cancer patient who died of myocardial infarction could be counted twice, once as a cancer death and once as a death

from myocardial infarct. In another example, for a death involving cerebral hemorrhage and coronary artery disease, the person could be counted as a death from cerebral hemorrhage and as a death from coronary artery disease. Multiple-cause tabulations even on a person basis are not additive; that is, the sum of deaths for persons with reports of heart disease and cancer will be greater than the sum of decedents with the conditions as the underlying cause.

Selecting a tabulation list

In the multiple-cause tabulations produced by NCHS, diseases and conditions counted are defined by the categories in selected-cause tabulation lists such as those recommended by WHO, or those routinely used by NCHS and recommended to states (72). Adopting a simple rule to count only one of the two or more conditions classifiable to the same group or subgroup takes care of the problem of repeated information within the same cause-of-death subgroup. For example, if Myocardial infarction (ICD–9 No. 410) and Angina pectoris (ICD 413) are jointly reported, these two terms are counted by NCHS only once under the broader rubric Ischemic heart disease (ICD 410–414). If Hypertensive heart disease (ICD 402) and Coronary sclerosis (ICD 414.0) are jointly reported, these terms are counted as Hypertensive heart disease (ICD 402) and Ischemic heart disease (ICD 410–414). However, these two forms of heart disease will be counted only once in the count of Diseases of the heart (ICD 390–398,402,400–429).

As Israel et al. pointed out, "counts of persons cannot necessarily be summed up to broader subgroups without unduplicating the multiple counts of the same person falling into the broader grouping" (73).

The count of malignant neoplasms as the cause of death in multiple-cause tabulations may present a special problem, because the various organs to which the cancer has metastasized are frequently reported. When the disease has spread and the primary site is not known, the medical certifier may report the cause of death in terms such as generalized carcinoma or carcinomatosis.

As a general rule, it is desirable to limit multiple-cause count of deaths of malignant neoplasms to the primary site of the disease. Information on the spread of the disease should be used only in the event that the primary site is not reported, in which case reported information on the secondary sites and the general spread of the disease will establish that the death was indeed due to a malignancy.

| 39 |

Suppressing terms representing mode of dying

Eliciting needed information on causes of death on the death certificate from the medical certifier has always been a problem. Developing a tabulation strategy for multiple-cause data can benefit from understanding the heterogeneous nature of diagnostic information on the death certificate. At the time of the medical examination, only certain signs and symptoms can be recorded if the disease process has not progressed to the stage where a diagnosis is possible, or if the clinical and pathological observations are inadequate or incomplete. A disease state may be described by physical signs alone (e.g., abscess, dermatitis, etc.), which may result from a variety of diseases. Or diseases may be referred to by a specific diagnostic term (e.g., pulmonary tuberculosis, measles, cancer of the breast, etc.). In general, physically descriptive and symptomatic terms are used to report diseases whose etiology is unknown or that cannot be diagnosed by the attending physician. Signs and symptoms may also be reported on the death certificate in addition to the disease itself.

As a result, expressions used to describe causes of morbidity and causes of death are a mixture of terms denoting symptoms, signs, and diseases. In addition, the medical certifier may report the mode or mechanisms of dying such as cardiac, renal, and respiratory failures [i.e., uninformative conditions involved in virtually all deaths (74)] as well as vague and ill-defined terms in describing diseases. Modes of dying are frequently reported on death certificates despite specific instructions on the death certificate to the medical certifier not to do so.

In developing multiple-cause tabulations, suppression of reported modes of dying is desirable because counting these terms inflates the count of diseases of the organ to which they relate. Information also may be repeated—for example, angina pectoris may be reported as anginal pain, coronary occlusion, or insufficiency. Or the death may be attributed to myocardial infarction. Some or all of these terms may be entered on the medical certificate in addition to the relevant disease that resulted in death. To count all of the manifestations of a disease for a death, therefore, is to duplicate the count of a particular disease entity. To tabulate everything reported on the death certificate is to count all diagnostic terms reported, which may differ considerably from a count of diseases.

Selected uses of multiple-cause data

The complexity of multiple-cause data has probably been a deterrent to its widespread use and its publication in routine statistical summaries, as suggested by Kochanek and Rosenberg (75). The most recent general statistical report on multiple causes in the United States, published by NCHS (76), was limited to fairly rudimentary comparisons of underlying cause and total reported causes. In contrast, multiple-cause data have been used in a large and growing number of special studies to augment traditional underlying cause analysis. The following summarizes some highlights from the NCHS report, and discusses additional analytical uses of multiple-cause data.

Ranking leading causes of death

The NCHS multiple-cause report (77) includes a comparison of underlying and multiple causes of death, and a comparison between the ranking of causes of death using the underlying and multiple-cause tabulations. Results show that most events such as suicide, homicide and accidents, and diseases such as cancer, acute myocardial infarction, hypertensive heart disease, and meningococcal infections, are well represented in the underlying cause of death statistics. In contrast, complications like septicemia and less lethal conditions such as nutritional deficiency, anemia, and hyperplasia of the prostate are frequently reported on death certificates but appear relatively infrequently in tabulations as the underlying cause of death.

As a consequence, shifts occur in the leading causes of death when ranked using multiple compared with underlying cause of death. As an underlying cause, accidents in 1978 ranked fourth, but they ranked sixth on the basis of all reported conditions (multiple cause). Arteriosclerosis advanced from eighth as an underlying cause to fourth as a multiple cause. The causes Bronchitis, emphysema and asthma, and septicemia—which did not appear among the 10 leading causes of death in the underlying cause tabulations—rank 8th and 9th, respectively, in multiple-cause tabulations, replacing cirrhosis of the liver and suicide, which occupied those positions in underlying cause tabulations.

Comparison of the 10 leading causes of death for 1993 shows that the same diseases appear in both lists, up to and including the 7th leading cause of death; however, the ranking of these diseases is not exactly the same in the two lists. The multiple-cause data attach slightly more importance to chronic obstructive lung diseases, pneumonia and influenza, and diabetes mellitus than the underlying cause data. Based on multiple-cause data for 1993, septicemia, atherosclerosis, and nephritis, nephritic syndrome and nephrosis appear as the 8th, 9th, and 10th leading causes of death, replacing HIV infection, suicide, and chronic liver diseases and cirrhosis of the liver as ranked in the underlying cause data.

Comparisons of multiple and underlying causes of death

Multiple-cause data add new dimensions to cause-of-death statistics. For example, person-based counts of diseases and conditions may provide a somewhat better indication of the prevalence of a disease or condition in the total population of deaths. As such, multiple-cause data give a more comprehensive view of causes of death than underlying cause statistics. For example, the number of deaths from Diseases of the heart as the underlying cause of death in 1993 is 743,460, whereas the number of death certificates with a report of some form of heart disease reported is 1,162,755, or 56 percent more than the number of deaths from heart disease as the underlying cause of death. In the case of multiple-cause data for heart disease, a bit of refinement is required because the death total for Diseases of the heart (in ICD–9) includes modes of dying such as heart failure and cardiac arrest without mention of a specific heart disease. Deleting Cardiac arrest (ICD–9 427.5) and Heart failure (ICD–9 428) reduces the number of those dying with a report of Diseases of the heart to 877,570, still 15 percent more than the number of deaths from Diseases of the heart as the underlying cause of death. However, the number of persons who had heart disease at the time of their death is substantially greater still based on 1993 National Mortality Followback Survey data.

With respect to renal diseases, the total count of persons who died with Nephritis, nephrotic syndrome and nephrosis (ICD–9 580–589) as a multiple cause is 124,160. When Renal failure (ICD–9 586) is excluded, the person-count of deaths from Nephritis, nephrotic syndrome and nephrosis drops to 52,316, a decrease of 58 percent, still more than twice the corresponding number of deaths from Nephritis, nephrotic syndrome and nephrosis as an underlying cause of death.

These findings demonstrate the analytical relevance of deleting modes of dying from underlying and multiple-cause counts of cardiovascular renal diseases until such time as the modes of dying are classified by WHO in the Symptoms and ill-defined causes of death instead of disease system chapters. Although the term "respiratory failure" is frequently reported on death certificates, this has no effect on the count of diseases of the respiratory system because Respiratory failure (ICD–9 799.1) is classified as a Symptom and ill-defined cause, not as a disease of the respiratory system.

Reports of secondary cancers and terms denoting generalized spread of the disease do not appear to have a substantial inflationary effect on the total count of deaths from malignant neoplasms. In 1993, a total of 596,385 deaths had a report on death certificates of malignant neoplasms. Of this total, the primary site was mentioned on

572,104 records. The difference of about 4 percent between these totals indicates that the primary site of cancer is well reported on deaths involving malignancies.

Because of the mortality coding rules for underlying cause of death, deaths from violence are rarely classified as a natural cause of death; in 1993, 98 percent or more of reported deaths from violence were attributed to accidents, homicides, and suicides as the underlying cause.

Of the leading causes of deaths, 92 percent of deaths for those with malignant neoplasms appear as such in underlying cause tabulations; 88 percent of deaths with mention of heart diseases are so classified as the underlying cause of death; but only 30 percent of deaths with a report of diabetes mellitus are charged to diabetes as the underlying cause of death.

Although the number of deaths involving tuberculosis and syphilis is now relatively small, a fairly large proportion of deaths involving these diseases is now reporting them as contributory causes of death within the multiple-cause data. Prior to 1940, when the joint-cause procedures were in use for classifying causes of death, virtually all infective diseases like tuberculosis and syphilis would have taken precedence over all other diseases, even if they were reported as a contributory cause of death.

A number of conditions are frequently reported on death certificates but appear relatively infrequently as the underlying cause of death. In 1993, hypertension (8 percent of records), nutritional deficiency (8 percent), septicemia (26 percent), and pneumonia (40 percent) were infrequently classified as the underlying cause of death in the records that mentioned these among the multiple causes of death.

Associations among causes of death

With respect to the criticism of underlying cause data that a single cause of death, no matter how selected, cannot adequately describe the medical circumstances surrounding death from chronic degenerative diseases where more than one disease is involved in the death, the cause of death may be represented by a composite of diseases formed by combining two or more diagnostic terms. For example, a death involving ischemic heart disease, diabetes, and prostate cancer could be attributed to a combination of these diagnostic terms, assuming their reporting was reasonably complete on death certificates.

Disease associations of many kinds can be revealed using multiple-cause data. Illustrative tabulations of such combinations of diseases are shown in Israel et al. (78). Tables showing associations can be useful for presenting data for diseases where death results from complications, such as Diabetes mellitus, but for which the ICD classification does not embed the complications in subcategories of the disease itself.

Assignment of a cause to death involving therapeutic misadventure, including untoward effects of operative procedures, has presented a problem in the past. With multiple-cause data, however, the problem is mitigated because the disease for which the treatment was given can be shown along with the effects of the therapeutic procedure. Associations can also be shown in relation to "expected associations," where the latter is estimated using joint probabilities, assuming independence.

Tabulation guidelines

Despite the value of multiple-cause data particularly for special studies, few routine multiple-cause tabulations have been produced by the United States or other countries. Further, relatively few guidelines are available for such tabulations. ICD–6 included a tentative suggestion for a table on multiple causes of death.

The question of what multiple-cause data should be routinely published is not simple, because the potential numbers of tabulations, particularly for associations, is very large, and larger still when cross-classified by standard demographic variables such as age and sex. Useful associations could include, for example, complications of selected diseases; diseases associated with therapeutic misadventures; and external causes of injury and poisonings cross-classified by nature of injury. To date, NCHS routinely produces tabulations for use as control totals with public-use microdata files. These annual multiple-cause tabulations are principally but not exclusively on a person-count basis (69).

In 1969, the group participating in WHO's Consultation on Multiple Cause Analysis produced a draft set of multiple-cause coding rules for trial use and suggested a format for some basic tables. This group also proposed a count of persons with reported specific diseases and conditions. The tabulation guidelines formulated by this group were presented to and received the commendation of WHO's Expert Committee on Health Statistics engaged in the preparatory work for ICD–9. However, the agendas for both the Ninth and the Tenth Decennial Revision conferences did not include the subject of multiple-cause coding procedures. In subsequent meetings of WHO's center heads, a number of proposals have been made for standardized multiple-cause tabulations, but these, too, have led to no official actions.

The absence of international guidelines for tabulating multiple-cause data may reflect the costs of manually coding multiple causes of death compared with underlying cause. It may also suggest that multiple-cause data most

fully reach their potential in special studies where they supplement traditional underlying cause data, providing a different and more comprehensive perspective on diseases and other causes of death. With the availability of multiple-cause data as a by-product of the computerized system for coding the underlying cause of death, cost is no longer a major issue. More and more countries will be producing multiple-cause data in years to come. Discussions of the most effective use of multiple-cause data would be valuable as additional countries routinely produce multiple-cause data.

In the United States, distribution of multiple-cause data is likely to continue to be principally in the form of electronic microdata files, which give users the maximum flexibility for research. Each of these annual files includes several sets of multiple-cause tabulations on both a condition as well as a person basis, although principally the latter. While the tabulations can and are used widely to respond to multiple-cause data requests, their principal use is as control totals for researchers.

Nevertheless, multiple-cause data as a by-product of securing the underlying cause of death can be analytically useful if properly understood and properly used. Moreover, the multiple causes of death reported, including the underlying cause, can theoretically give a more complete view of the cause of death, because frequently more than one disease or condition is involved in a death. Additional nonstatistical uses of multiple-cause data will be discussed in a later chapter.

CHAPTER 6

Comparability and Accuracy of
Cause-of-death Statistics

ICD has had a major role in promoting comparability among nations by providing a common classification, methods for classifying causes of death, and rules for coding causes of death that can be used by all countries for tabulation and analysis of morbidity and mortality statistics. However, having common guidelines does not ensure that resulting statistics will be comparable. This chapter discusses different aspects of comparability and accuracy of cause-of-death statistics. Problems of data comparability may arise from differences in diagnostic methods and reporting, and from differences in terminology among countries where, for example, the same term may mean different things. In addition, historically, variations in coding practice and interpretation of international coding rules contributed to differences in resultant statistics. Different comparability issues arise when comparing cause-of-death statistics over time. Comparability problems may result from ICD revisions that affect the classification, coding rules, and design of the international death certificate. Other comparability differences may result from changes in diagnostic terminology and from the introduction of new diagnostic technologies such as the introduction of computer-assisted tomography (CAT scan) and magnetic resonance imaging (MRI), which resulted in changes in disease ascertainment.

Even if data were comparable among countries and population groups, questions of validity and accuracy of the reported cause of death remain. How well does the physician's medical certification reflect the medical history and, ultimately, the medical facts of death? Can accuracy and validity be assessed and measured?

Finally, how can cause-of-death statistics be improved? Are there practical methods for impressing upon physicians the importance of accurate medical certification? Can physicians be educated and trained to provide better certifications of cause of death? Assuming so, through what kind of modalities? Are feedback methods available to alert physicians to poor certification practice and to reinforce good certification practice?

This chapter summarizes knowledge about comparability and accuracy of cause of death. For comparability, it

discusses some issues of comparability among countries and over time. In terms of accuracy, the chapter describes methodologies used to assess accuracy, and available statistical indicators for monitoring data quality for causes of death. Finally, the chapter reviews efforts and approaches to improving the quality of cause-of-death statistics.

Comparability

The value of any statistic lies in the ability to compare data, be it to compare data from two or more sources for a particular period of time, or to compare data from the same source over a period of time. For these purposes, the data from all sources need to be as comparable as possible. Although a uniform classification is essential, other factors that are of importance in producing comparable data include use of acceptable and relatively comparable medical terminology, use of a common source document, proper completion of the source document, and uniform interpretation and application of coding rules.

The importance of a common classification was stressed by William A. King, Chief Statistician for Vital Statistics, U.S. Census Office, who stated in the preface to ICD–1, "It is much more important that deaths reported in the same terms shall everywhere be compiled under the same titles than the assignment be absolutely correct" (21).

The five general rules proposed by Bertillon were meant to standardize coding procedures. Despite international recognition of ICD at the beginning of the 20th century, application of these rules was not obligatory, and use of ICD among nations was recognized to be highly variable until ICD–6, when WHO Regulations No. 1 was promulgated. Although the selection rules used by countries varied greatly, there was general agreement on certain points. Most countries gave precedence to violent deaths, infectious diseases, and fatal diseases, in the order named.

Although the mandatory nature of Regulations No. 1 helps promote uniformity in mortality statistics, this alone is no assurance that comparability will be achieved. For example, it cannot be assumed that all national offices will keep in step on coding practices unless they all use the same computerized coding system, like ACME, and indeed the same version of ACME, because the automated system has been modified a number of times since implementation of ICD–10. Comparability questions may also arise when data for the same area are compared over time, especially if changes have occurred in the classification system or coding methods.

Comparability of data between countries

At the request of the Commission for Revision of the International List of Causes of Death in 1929, the U.S. Bureau of the Census prepared 1,032 medical certificates, each involving two to five diseases or conditions, together with other relevant data (52). These cases were submitted to the national statistical offices of various countries with the request that they be classified according to the selection principles currently employed in those offices. Eighteen countries responded to the request.

The average agreement among the countries in the selection of the primary cause of death was relatively low (57.5 percent). The agreement between individual countries ranged from about 90 percent to 32 percent. By cause of death, the highest average agreement was in the assignment of cases involving cancer. The average agreement was low in cases involving diseases such as anemia, cerebral hemorrhage and cerebral embolism, diseases of the prostate, and alcoholism. Because the cases included in the study were selected to characterize joint-cause classification problems, results of the comparisons could not be used as correction factors. However, they did indicate the kind of differences that can result from the lack of uniformity in the rules, or in the interpretation of the rules, for selecting the primary cause of death.

Since then, numerous similar studies that have been conducted essentially confirmed intercountry variation in manual application of the mortality coding rules. For example, in 1958, a comparison deck of 6,000 medical certificates—2,000 each from Canada, England and Wales, and the United States—were coded by the three national offices (79). The same deck and the code assignments were then sent to the WHO Center for Classification of Diseases in London, and a meeting was held to discuss the results of the coding exercise. Many of the disagreements arose because of differences in interpreting the rules or in the manner in which the causes of death were reported. The group worked out interpretations acceptable to the three countries and to the WHO center.

The same kind of exercise was conducted by the WHO Regional Office for Europe (80). Samples of coded death certificates from Denmark, Finland, and Germany were sent to the WHO Center for Classification of Diseases in London. Results of this study showed that coding differences did not have a great effect on death rates for arteriosclerotic and degenerative heart disease, but they did have an important influence on the death rate for other causes of death such as vascular lesions of the central nervous system, rheumatic heart disease, and bronchitis.

This study of accuracy of coding causes of death and comparability of national statistics on causes of death was extended to include Czechoslovakia, Denmark, Finland, the Netherlands, Sweden, and the United Kingdom. A sample of 1,000 death certificates in English was circulated to the participating countries for coding according to the normal national practice. The code assignments were then compared with the corresponding assignments made by the WHO center. The study showed considerable disagreement between individual countries and between these countries and the WHO center in selecting and coding the underlying cause of death. Much of the disagreement was because ICD coding provisions had apparently been ignored.

In another study conducted by the Euro Office of WHO (81), standard case histories of cardiovascular diseases were sent to six countries—Austria, Bulgaria, Czechoslovakia, Federal Republic of Germany, France, and the United Kingdom. After the group of clinicians filled out the medical certificates from information contained in the clinical abstracts, the national office coded the underlying cause of death. The study showed that there was less variation from coding practice than from variations attributable to medical certification practices. This indicated a need to clarify the meaning of the "underlying cause of death" and the correct way in which to complete the medical certificate of death.

Comparability over time

When revisions are made in the disease classification or in coding rules, changes can occur in assigning deaths to ICD categories, potentially creating discontinuities in mortality trends and patterns. These discontinuities can be measured by coding death certificates (or a sample thereof) for a particular year by the old and new disease classifications, employing the coding rules used with the respective classifications. The ratio of the number of deaths assigned to the various rubrics of the respective classifications can be calculated and is called a "comparability ratio." Alternatively, the proportion of deaths in each old category assigned to each of the new rubrics can be calculated, and vice versa. Either method permits the construction of estimated frequencies for comparable rubrics of the old or new classification and provides a bridge between the two.

The *Registrar-General's Statistical Review of England and Wales* for 1938 and 1939 is devoted to cause-of-death tabulations made according to ICD–4 and ICD–5 coded by the respective rules in effect (82). Also presented in that report are data on deaths classified to the various disease categories in the three-year period, 1936 through 1938, by the old selection method and by the certifiers' order of preference.

Because the old selection rules patterned after Bertillon had not been seriously modified since their adoption in 1901, comparability of tabulation is presumed to have been maintained from 1901 to 1927. In 1927, the selection rules were replaced by the opinion of the medical certifier as expressed by the order in the statement of causes of death. Comparability studies such as those referred to above have been made after each subsequent ICD revision.

The first comparability study in the United States was made by Dunn and Shackley (83). This study traced each term in the tabular list from ICD–4 to ICD–5. Analysis of cause-of-death assignments of mortality data for 1940 made by ICD–4 and ICD–5 showed the number of deaths that were transferred to the different rubrics of the international list and the reasons for the transfer, that is, whether brought about by revision of the classification or by revision of the coding rules.

As in England and Wales, comparability was greatly affected in the United States when the certifiers' statement of the underlying cause of death, rather than the coding rules, was accepted as the basis for classifying the underlying cause of death. Faust and Dolman (84,85) published comparability reports from ICD–5 to ICD–7. Klebba prepared comparability ratios in connection with the Eighth Revision of the International Classification of Diseases Adapted for Indexing Hospital Records (ICDA–8) and ICD–9 (86,87).

The most recent comparability study for the United States—between ICD–9 and ICD–10—was carried out by Robert Anderson and his colleagues at NCHS using a large sample of records processed mostly by using automated coding (54). Automation, which greatly facilitates studies of comparability between ICD revisions, must increasingly be used due to WHO's continuous updating process implemented with ICD–10. Comparability studies will be needed to evaluate the impact of these continuous changes in the classification.

Comparability studies are also important for evaluating the quantitative impact of changing from manual to automated coding. A number of countries, including Australia and England, conducted such comparability studies when they implemented automated cause-of-death coding (88,89).

Continuous expansion of ICD from 179 rubrics in 1900 to about 8,000 categories in 1999 makes it difficult to follow the trend in mortality for many disease categories

across revisions. However, it is possible to analyze mortality over long periods in two ways: 1) starting with broad rubrics and going backward by judiciously grouping data into comparable categories combined with information from various comparability studies, and 2) limiting the analyses to the period during which the data are comparable within revision periods. Comparability ratios for various periods make it possible to bridge gaps observed in trend data unless irresolvable discontinuities are present. Comparability studies, and more specifically comparability ratios, are most relevant to the immediate years of transition to a new revision, because some ratios actually change over time as a result of changes in medical terminology, in the mix of detailed titles that may comprise a broader tabulation category, and in the demographic mix of the population (54). Detailed statistical methods for bridging revisions are described in recent reports by Hoyert and others (90).

When discontinuities in trend result from ICD revisions, it may be possible to reconstruct the trend for the period prior to the revision by a judicious grouping of the components that were subdivided in the revision. However, any revision change that affects comparability of data is, at best, inconvenient and annoying. Not being able to adjust or account for the breaks in trend can be frustrating, but worse still is not to recognize the effects of revision changes and interpret them as real differences. For the statistician, frequent revisions can create problems in analyzing trend data. On the other hand, infrequent revisions, as between ICD–9 and ICD–10, cause difficulties for nonstatistical users such as those concerned with medical reimbursements.

Other factors

The historic comparability of mortality data is affected by more than statistical practice and ICD changes. Medical practice and technology can also affect comparability even if classification systems remain constant (91). Medical terminology can change in ways that can profoundly influence mortality trends. In the late 1960s, the introduction of new terminology for chronic respiratory diseases resulted in major declines in asthma, bronchitis, and emphysema, with compensating increases in a newly introduced, nonspecific term, "Chronic obstructive pulmonary disease without mention of asthma, bronchitis, and emphysema." The introduction of other new terms, such as SIDS in the 1970s and AIDS in the 1980s, also markedly affected cause-of-death statistics in other categories (92).

Changes in diagnostic technology can also affect trends. Introduction of the CAT scanner appears to have been associated with sharp increases in brain cancer mortality, which likely represented changes in ascertainment rather than incidence (93).

| 45 |

Comparability can also be affected by changes in data collection forms. When the United States introduced the revision of the standard certificate of death with an additional fourth line in Part I of the medical certification portion of the death certificate in 1989, an abrupt increase occurred in a number of causes of death, notably diabetes, with compensating declines for other causes of death (94).

Accuracy of cause of death

A considerable body of literature deals with the quality of cause-of-death statistics (95,96). This is all to the good, because the accuracy and validity of cause-of-death statistics is frequently challenged, paradoxically often by members of the medical community whose responsibility it is to complete medical certifications as carefully and thoughtfully as possible.

It is desirable to have on hand information on validity to provide empirically based responses to such challenges, and to supplement these with the statistical perspectives that 1) mortality data are the best available disease-specific information despite their limitations, and 2) having quantitative estimates of bias or error provide the basis for properly qualifying available statistical estimates.

Types of validation studies

Some studies of validity are concerned with measuring the precision of clinical diagnoses. Others are related to ascertaining the validity of cause of death for specific diseases or groups of diseases such as cancer, cardiovascular diseases, cerebrovascular diseases, tuberculosis, diabetes, chronic bronchopulmonary diseases, etc.

These validation studies often vary in their objectives, methodologies, and criteria of matches and mismatches. In general, three standards have been used for comparisons with diagnoses reported on death certificates. These are: 1) autopsy records, 2) clinical records, and 3) all available medical information, that is, the combination of 1) and 2) and data from other sources such as lay informants, physicians' visits, disease registers, etc. In each of these approaches, source data are used to ascertain the cause of death (or the underlying cause of death) independent of the information on the death certificate, and, in turn, are compared with the statement of the cause of death on the death certificate.

Autopsies have long been used for confirming clinical diagnoses and have served as a valuable teaching tool. However, for measurement purposes, the proportion of cases that come to autopsy must be recognized as being relatively small. In addition to the problem of numbers,

autopsy cases are highly selective. Only the more difficult diagnostic problems, cases of unusual clinical interest, or those of medical legal concern, are subject to postmortem examination. The biased nature of autopsy data has been discussed by Berkson (97), Mainland (98), and Cornfield (99).

Studies show varying lack of correspondence between the causes of death entered on death certificates and information found in clinical records or autopsy protocols. However, these studies, involving as they do the reconstruction of case histories by persons other than the attending physician, are different from an attending physician's evaluation of clinical findings in light of postmortem reports. Many records are extremely sketchy, especially those cases in which the patient was admitted to the hospital "dead on arrival."

Absolute precision of diagnoses cannot be expected. Despite continuing medical progress, differences will always exist in diagnostic acumen between medical practitioners. The most that can be expected of cause-of-death statistics is that they reflect as accurately as possible current medical opinion concerning causes of death based on information available at the time of death.

Statistical indicators of quality

An in-depth understanding of the validity of cause of death reported by the certifying physician best results from comparing death records with the most precise available assessment of the decedents' cause of death and the factors leading to it based on a variety of information.

In contrast, a general statistical assessment is possible using a variety of indicators. One of the most common such statistical measures is the percentage of deaths for which the underlying cause was assigned to the category "Symptoms and ill-defined conditions." Similarly, the number and proportion of deaths assigned to modes of dying such as cardiac arrest, pulmonary arrest, coma, and the many other terms representing symptoms rather than diseases, can provide yardsticks for measuring quality.

Another indicator is the percentage of deaths assigned to causes of death for which the ICD number ends with the 4th-digit 0.9, which is generally used to classify a diagnostic term to an "unspecified" or "other and unspecified" category. When a diagnosis is assigned to a category ending with the 4th-digit 0.9, it suggests that the diagnostic term was not sufficiently precise to be assigned to a more explicit condition in the 4th-digit range 0.0 through 0.8.

Another statistical approach to measuring quality of medical certification is to determine which coding rules were invoked by the mortality medical coder or automated system to select the underlying cause of death. The coding rule that suggests a relatively correctly completed certification is the "General Rule" or "General Principle," which applies when the condition reported on the lowest-used line of Part I can etiologically give rise to all the conditions reported above it, and, therefore, can be designated the "tentative" underlying cause of death. The tentative underlying cause may be subsequently modified by taking into account other conditions in Part I or Part II of the death certificate. If the General Rule applies, it can be symptomatic (but no guarantee) of a good certification.

Another approach for assessing quality uses multiple-cause data. Assuming that the number of conditions reported on a death certificate reflects the care with which the cause of death was reported, the number of causes on each certificate can be tabulated, and the average number of conditions per certificate, for example, or the percent distribution of the number of conditions, can be used as an indicator.

The great value of statistical indicators of quality is to provide comparative assessments of certification quality over time and among geographic areas.

Improving the quality of medical certification of cause of death

Studies of validity and reliability have, thus far, not provided unequivocal results regarding the accuracy of diagnoses on death certificates. Nevertheless, the preponderance of evidence on both a qualitative and quantitative basis suggests that improvements in medical certification of death can and should be undertaken. To this end, a number of approaches have been taken historically to address these concerns. These have included *inter alia* improving instructions for death certificates, developing training materials on medical certification, and promoting cause-of-death querying programs.

Encouraging querying

Although civil registration and vital statistics systems can do little about improving the diagnostic acumen of medical practitioners, much can be done to improve the completeness and quality of cause-of-death statements on the death certificate.

One of the early concerns in reporting cause of death was the use of indefinite and ill-defined medical terminology by medical certifiers in completing cause of death on death certificates. A list of such terms was published in every ICD published by the U.S. Bureau of the Census starting in 1900. Vital registrars were encouraged to familiarize themselves with these undesirable terms so that when such

terms were received as the sole statement of cause of death, they were to return the death certificate to the medical certifier for further information. This process of certificate review and quality assessment, including communication between the vital statistics office and certifying physician, is called "querying."

Local registration officials or state vital statistics programs review medical certifications to promote quality assurance of cause-of-death reporting (100,101). Querying is often handled by expert medical coders, who evaluate the cause-of-death report using querying guidelines prepared at the national level and adapted for state and local use (102). Under these guidelines, cause-of-death statements that are either incomplete (e.g., cancer without specification of site) or uninformative (cardiac arrest) result in communication with the physician to obtain additional information or to clarify ambiguities.

Querying is known to be one of the most effective ways to improve the quality of medical certification. Benefits derive from the medical certifier's awareness that the information is being scrutinized for quality and will be used for statistical purposes. Improved certifications also result because of the educational function of providing feedback and instruction to the medical certifier on proper procedures, lessons that may contribute to better certifications in the future (103). In states that have implemented strong querying programs, the percentage of records that need to be queried and modified gradually drops over time.

The importance of querying statements of cause was recognized early in the history of the U.S. Death Registration Area. The Bureau of the Census sent queries directly to the medical certifiers by mail until the 1930s, when the function was shifted to state vital statistics offices. This was in addition to queries already made by the state vital statistics offices.

Prior to 1949, medical certifiers were queried primarily for more specific information on the cause of death when vague and ill-defined terms were reported. With the revision of the joint-cause selection procedure in 1949, this approach became inadequate. In addition to what was to be reported, the order in which the causes were given in the underlying cause sequence and the relationships between them became important. Querying, as a process, became highly complex.

The National Office of Vital Statistics (predecessor agency to NCHS) queried about 10,000 medical certifications annually (i.e., less than 1 percent) until the 1950s, when this practice was discontinued because of cost. At that time, about one-quarter of the certificates were candidates for querying because of errors in the order or the arrangement of the reported causes of death.

| 47 |

In the late 1980s, most states had some level of querying, which was required under the provisions of federal-state cooperative agreements that provide NCHS with vital statistics information. However, at state urging in the early 1990s, NCHS relaxed the cause-of-death querying requirement in the annual agreement between NCHS and the states. In the early 2000s, about 4 percent of total U.S. death records were queried about cause of death (102).

Guidelines for developing electronic death registration systems suggest the possibility of incorporating querying in the system, which future development of automated coding software may facilitate. NCHS continues to maintain a minimal level of querying for selected causes of death, principally those that are public health threats such as dangerous infectious diseases (e.g., cholera and plague) and vaccine-preventable diseases (e.g., diphtheria). NCHS no longer carries out a random program of querying, but it encourages states to continue a minimal level of querying as part of mortality statistics quality assurance. As electronic death registration continues to develop and be implemented, it may be possible to incorporate querying in the electronic medical certification process by interactively asking questions about incomplete and uninformative statements on cause of death and seeking immediate, online modification. Further, positive feedback could take the form of commending certifiers for informative cause-of-death statements.

Workshops on improving cause-of-death statistics

How to improve the accuracy of cause-of-death reporting was addressed in two NCHS-sponsored workshops, one in 1989 (104) and the other in 1991 (105). The discussions and recommendations covered a range of subjects including education of physicians, possible revision of the medical certificate format, and development of a model quality assessment program. The workshops were more formal than numerous past discussions on the same subject and well structured, drawing attendance from major professional organizations, federal agencies, and state civil registration systems.

Several recommendations of the workshops were implemented. Notably, they included: 1) simplified and convenient instructions for physicians, 2) exhibits on death certificate information for medical professional meetings, 3) improvements in death certificate instructions, 4) online tutorials and instructional materials, and 5) explicit statements in research articles and publications that attribute the source of cause-of-death statistics to diagnostic statements made by certifying physicians on death certificates. Other recommendations addressed what types of education and training would be most effective for

new physicians as well as those longer in practice. Some of the recommendations amplified existing but sporadic practice; others were innovative and, in a number of cases, practical to implement. Following is a brief summary of some of the approaches recommended to improve medical certification on death certificates.

Instructional materials

Instructional materials addressed to medical certifiers were developed and improved over the years by WHO, NCHS, and the states. In 1900, the first "physician's handbook" was issued in the United States titled, *Physicians' Pocket Reference to the International List of Causes of Death*. The sole purpose of this pocket edition was to obtain cause-of-death statements in precise and definite terms. ICD titles were reproduced in this publication, and those titles or parts of the title representing specific disease entities stated in acceptable terminology were shown in boldfaced type. In addition to the preferred titles in boldface, the indefinite or otherwise undesirable terms were shown in italics. The rest of the pocket reference was devoted to reasons why certain terms were undesirable. This material remained substantially the same through eight revisions. In the Eighth Revision of the Pocket Reference, ICD titles were reproduced without the boldfaced type, italics, or instructions.

The 1938 handbook represented a major change in purpose and content. The *Physicians' Handbook of Birth and Death Registration* took up, in addition to the subject of medical certification, problems of geographic and personal particulars in connection with birth certificates, death certificates, and fetal death reports. It described the history of vital registration and provided the definition of rates and other indexes. A selected bibliography of vital statistics was shown as well as some vital statistics. The handbook also included an abbreviated ICD to fill the gap for coders while the 1939 revision of the International List was being prepared for publication. The 1938 Physicians' Handbook became a standard reference for students in schools of public health. The 1948 revision reverted to the barest essentials that the physicians had to know about filling out birth and death certificates and reports of fetal death.

WHO issued its first booklet on *Medical Certificate of Causes of Death* in 1952 to accompany ICD–6. Subsequent editions were published to accompany ICD–7, ICD–8, and ICD–9. In the same series, WHO published *Amplification of the Medical Certificate of Cause of Death*, which dealt with inquiries to medical certifiers in relation to incomplete or vague statements reported on the medical certificate.

The *Physicians' Handbook on Birth and Death Registration*, or its equivalent, is a reference source for physicians and funeral directors in the United States on registration procedures, including the medical certification of causes of death. NCHS periodically issues a revision of this handbook. The most recent revision has separate handbooks for physicians and for coroners and medical examiners (106).

As a supplement to the Physicians' Handbook, a film strip on medical certification of causes of death was prepared in the 1950s for training medical certifiers. Hospitals and medical societies were the intended audience for this homemade production of a 35 mm film and phonograph record. The film strip drew considerable interest. Subsequently, a color movie was produced in which the uniformed Surgeon General introduced the subject, and a commercial announcer gave the narration. A copy of the film was sent to every state vital statistics office, and several copies were placed in CDC's film library so that it would be available to any interested person. An effective presentation could supplement the film with a knowledgeable instructor, who could respond to questions.

Subsequently, a videocassette on death registration was produced and issued, one oriented to medical examiners and coroners and the other to physicians. At that time, videos were more convenient than films that required projectors.

In the early 1990s, NCHS prepared instructions for physicians on completing death certificates in the format of a laminated plastic card, 8.5 by 11 inches, under the CDC logo. The laminated cards provided not only instructions on completing medical certification but also examples of properly completed cause-of-death statements. Two cards were prepared, one for deaths from natural causes (available from http://www.cdc.gov/nchs/data/dvs/blue_form.pdf) and the other for deaths from accidents, injuries, and poisonings (available from http://www.cdc.gov/nchs/data/dvs/red_form.pdf). The latter was developed with coroners and medical examiners in mind, because they prepare most of the certificates due to external causes. The laminated cards have been highly popular in the United States, having been widely distributed by state vital statistics offices to hospitals and physicians throughout the country. The laminated cards have also been used as models in other countries.

Exhibits for medical professional society meetings

Another outgrowth of the workshops to improve cause-of-death information are exhibits. The exhibits, which have been presented at selected professional medical society meetings, are staffed jointly by NCHS and state vital statistics staff and have been well received. The medical professional meetings have included those concerned with family practice, heart diseases, cancer, minority medical groups, geriatrics, coroners, and medical examiners.

Expanded instructions on death certificates

Vital records in the United States are usually modified once every 10 years (48). The revisions take into account changes in legal requirements, social conventions, technology, and research needs and interests. The process for revising certificates involves a broad range of stakeholders, including state and federal vital registration officials, researchers, academicians, statisticians, etc. The revision of the death certificate designed for implementation in 2003 (107) includes far more detailed instructions, listed separately for the physician completing the cause-of-death section and for the funeral director who is responsible both for providing the demographic information and for filing the completed certificate with civil registration authorities. This latest revised death certificate is designed to have three pages: a top sheet of removable instructions to the physician, the actual certificate in the center, and a bottom page of removable instructions for the funeral director.

Electronic death registration

Beginning in the late 1990s, NCHS, working closely with the National Association for Public Health Statistics and Information Systems and with the states as well as the Social Security Administration (SSA), initiated a project to evaluate the feasibility of electronic death registration (108). The SSA's interest focuses on death clearance, that is, on early and accurate notification of deaths for termination of benefit payments. The states' interest focuses on improving the efficiency and effectiveness of vital registration, and on the receipt of more timely and accurate information on vital events.

The electronic death registration project was initiated at a time when the feasibility of electronic registration had been successfully demonstrated for births, in which more than 90 percent of events are registered electronically. It was believed that electronic death registration could benefit from the experience with electronic birth registration, in particular by establishing standards at the outset on overall system design, minimum item content, item presentation in an electronic format, and secure electronic transmission of confidential information. When the project was initiated in 1996, only one state, New Hampshire, had a working electronic death registration system, but it was essentially an electronic adaptation of a paper system and, therefore, did not take full advantage of many potential electronic functionalities, including interactive edits, tutorials, and potential linkage with processing software.

Electronic death registration is now an integral component of the federal-state program to "re-engineer" the national vital registration system in a way that not only takes greater advantage of electronic capabilities but can be integrated with other statistical and nonstatistical systems.

For the electronic death registration system, NCHS created a standard module on medical certification of death—including detailed instructions on completing cause of death—which reflects the revised certificate of death. These detailed instructions have subsequently been incorporated in specifications for developing systems (108).

Web-based training

The rapid development of the Internet has had major implications for data quality. A number of efforts have been undertaken to develop online materials specifically directed to improving the quality of medical certification. For example, the National Association of Medical Examiners and others have developed online, interactive information on how to complete the medical certification of death (106). In addition, NCHS has created electronic versions of the laminated plastic cards and the handbooks (106).

Training and education

Almost every meeting on the subject of improving medical certification of causes of death seems to conclude with the suggestion for a course on medical certification to be offered to medical students. Because this is such a logical and simple solution to a difficult problem, the proposal is usually accepted without debate. A major problem, however, is that students in their third or fourth year of medical study, the period most suitable for such a course, have limited time and interest to devote to a topic other than clinical medicine.

Other recommendations would include questions on medical certification procedures in national board examinations and offer training courses on medical certification to interns and residents as well as in Continuing Medical Education (CME) (106). Board examination questions are a possibility, but courses during hospital internship or residency raise questions of how such a program would be managed. CME courses have been successfully implemented in recent years and can be highly effective, especially if conducted by medical examiners familiar with death certification.

Redesigning the death certificate

One of the recommendations of the workshops concerned possible revision of the present medical certificate, that is, to reverse the order of the sequence of events in Part I of the medical certificate form.

The 1900 medical certificate form requested the "cause of death" and the "contributory cause of death." Obtaining proper responses to these direct questions on causes of death was difficult. In subsequent revisions, minor changes were made in the wording of these items, with little success. In 1925, Stevenson introduced the proposal

that started with the immediate cause of death and went backward in time, ending with the underlying cause of death. This was adopted as the international medical certificate form in 1948.

For ICD–8, the Statistical Office of the Federal Republic of Germany expressed dissatisfaction with this reporting procedure that went backward in time and proposed instead that the sequence of events in Part I of the medical certificate be reversed. The import of this suggestion is to report first the underlying cause of death, followed by the resulting causes and ending with the immediate cause of death. If the medical certifier is able to state first the underlying cause of death, there would be no need to report the subsequent causes, much less the immediate cause of death. In effect, this is basically the procedure employed in the 1900 medical certificate form which proved so unsatisfactory.

The recommendation to evaluate a "reversed" medical certification was undertaken by NCHS in the 1990s. A research team designed a study in which medical case studies were submitted to a sample of physicians. After instruction, physicians—divided into groups—were to complete medical certifications for these cases using different formats, including the standard format and a reverse format. Because of the small size of the sample, the results are suggestive rather than definitive, but they indicate that the reported underlying cause did not differ significantly between the two formats. However, the number of reported causes was slightly larger using the reverse format (109).

Thus, the two workshops inspired a number of initiatives to improve cause-of-death reporting. They heightened awareness among state registration officials of the importance of accurate medical certification, and they resulted in both short- and long-term proposals for addressing the outstanding problems. Given the changing technological environment and continuing changes in the vital registration system, periodically convening a workshop to review the status of quality of cause of death, assess methods that have been beneficial in promoting quality, and propose new methods in light of changing technology, vital records, and medical practice may be prudent.

Given the importance of the national mortality database for tracking the nation's health and conducting health research, a major national initiative to reach all physicians would be required. Such an effort would probably require the endorsement of major medical professional groups, state registration officials, and a high-level spokesperson representing the U.S. Public Health Service.

CHAPTER 7
Related Health Classifications

Development of ICD during the past century has been accompanied and influenced by a proliferation of uses, but especially by expanding the use of ICD from statistical purposes into other areas, principally indexing hospital records and medical reimbursement. At the same time, other classification systems have been developed for various medical specialties and administrative purposes. Recognizing these parallel developments, WHO has attempted, to some extent, to embrace these developments, harmonize them as much as possible with ICD, and bring them into WHO's larger family of classifications. The expansion of nonstatistical uses has also influenced the content of the classification itself. This chapter briefly reviews the development of parallel classifications and the way in which they relate to ICD.

Expanded use of ICD for indexing hospital records

Through ICD–6, the decennial revisions of ICD were sufficient to meet the needs of both science and the broader health care community. However, shortly after the introduction of ICD–6, the shortcomings of ICD for nonstatistical purposes were becoming ever more apparent to users in that community. In 1952, the U.S. National Committee on Vital and Health Statistics appointed a study group to prepare an adaptation of ICD for indexing hospital records. The draft classification that this group prepared was subjected to a rigorous test in a comparative study conducted by AHA and cosponsored by the American Association of Medical Record Librarians (110). In this study, the versions of the *Standard Nomenclature of Diseases and Operations* (SNDO) of AMA and ICD in place at that time were used in a parallel test to see whether SNDO or ICD was more effective for retrieving specified diagnostic data from hospital records.

The study showed that 1) ICD could be used efficiently for disease indexing in hospitals, 2) coding and posting time was less with ICD than with SNDO, 3) there was a higher degree of consistency and reliability of coding with ICD than with SNDO, and 4) more records pertinent to the request were likely to be found using ICD rather than

SNDO. However, in accomplishing this, more nonpertinent records were also likely to be drawn from the files.

The study group suggested that ICD could be an effective tool for hospital use if the following changes could be made: 1) creation of finer subdivisions of certain categories to permit identification of specific diagnoses frequently requested of the record room, 2) deletion of residual categories involving ill-defined terminology, 3) deletion of all nonspecific or ambiguous descriptions of diseases, 4) substitution of the classification of mental disorders of the American Psychiatric Association for the section on Psychoses, Psychoneuroses and Behavioral Disorders, and 5) addition of a classification of operative and therapeutic procedures.

Following the evaluation study, a group representing major users of ICD in the hospital field consolidated their experiences in making further modifications of ICD for hospital indexing. An operation and treatment classification was also developed and incorporated in the first edition of the *International Classification of Diseases Adapted for Indexing of Hospital Records by Diseases and Operations*, published by the U.S. Public Health Service as a national adaptation of the Seventh Revision of the ICD with increased detail that was more responsive to the needs of health administration, including indexing hospital records (111).

After the United States' adaptation of the Seventh Revision of the ICD to provide a diagnostic cross-index for hospitals in the United States, similar adaptations were made by Sweden and Israel. PAHO published a Spanish translation of the U.S. adaptation of the Seventh Revision for use by hospitals in Latin American countries.

The Eighth Revision Conference noted that ICD–8 had been devised with hospital indexing needs in mind and considered that the classification would be suitable for hospital use in some countries but perhaps not adequate for diagnostic indexing in others. The conference therefore recommended that WHO prepare an adaptation of the revised classification that would be more widely applicable to indexing of hospital records.

Because this recommendation was not implemented, the U.S. Public Health Service asked a group of consultants to study ICD–8 to ascertain its suitability for indexing hospital records and for coding hospital morbidity data in the United States. The group recommended that additional detail be provided for these purposes. AHA was then requested to develop needed adaptation proposals. Its Advisory Committee to the Central Office on the ICDA prepared an adaptation that was published by NCHS—the *Eighth Revision of the International Classification of Diseases Adapted for Use in the United States*—for coding diagnostic data for official morbidity and mortality statistics, and for preparing diagnostic cross-indexes in hospitals in the United States (112).

In view of the growing use of ICD for creating diagnostic cross-indexes, adaptation of ICD–9 for that purpose was proposed. The proposal was adopted but not implemented. However, the United States produced an adapted version of the Ninth Revision, the *U.S. Clinical Modification of ICD–9* (ICD–9–CM) for use in health care settings, for indexing medical records, and for medical reimbursement (113). Other countries including Canada and Australia have developed their own adaptations of ICD designed to better meet their own needs for medical reimbursement and records indexing. For reimbursement, the codes of the ICD adaptation (or the ICD) are translated into Diagnostic Related Groups or DRGs, which take other factors into account and determine the amount of payment to be made for reimbursement to health care providers such as hospitals or physicians. Although preserving the overarching structure of ICD, the "clinical modifications" of ICD are much more detailed than the official WHO version of the classification. Moreover, decennial revisions were insufficient for health care purposes, and an annual updating process for the clinical modification was instituted in the United States to keep the classification abreast of advances in medical science and address largely nonstatistical needs.

Family of classifications

Because of the increasing uses of ICD for a variety of purposes, WHO called a conference in 1979 at Taormina, Sicily, even before ICD–9 came into use, to consider the long-term implications for ICD. Out of this conference evolved the concept of the basic ICD as the core of a "family" of associated classifications. Some suggested that WHO experiment with alternative structures, possibly triaxial, for the core classification. In a family of classifications, ICD could be the core classification with a series of modules, some hierarchically related and others of a supplemental nature. After some study and discussions with WHO Collaborating Centers, the concept of a family of classifications was developed. This scheme was

subsequently reconsidered and revised by the WHO Expert Committee on Health Statistics in 1987 (17).

The conference noted an example of the linkage of the ICD family of classifications in the medico-social and multidimensional assessment of the elderly in relation to health and activities of daily living as well as social and physical environment. It was shown that effective information could be obtained by the use of ICD and the *International Classification of Impairments, Disabilities and Handicaps*, especially by use of the code proposed in Chapter XXI of ICD–10.

Systematized Nomenclature of Pathology and Medicine

To meet the needs of pathologists, the College of American Pathologists issued the *Systematized Nomenclature of Pathology* (SNOP) in 1965 (114). SNOP classified pathological observations according to topography, morphology, etiology, and function. Each of these classifications, independent from the others, used 4-digit codes with a letter prefix for identifying the axis of classification in a hierarchical structure. This arrangement was carried through successively in the topographic and morphological classifications. Because of the amount of detail involved, parts of the etiologic and function codes could not be collapsed conveniently into homogeneous groupings. The purpose of SNOP was to make the retrieval of case records, tissue slides, photographs, etc., efficient.

The *Systematized Nomenclature of Medicine* (SNOMED) originated as an extension and adaptation of SNOP to provide a classification for clinical medicine (114,115). SNOMED has expanded greatly over time to reflect different medical fields. One of the milestones in integration and expansion efforts for SNOMED was the release of the *Systematized Nomenclature of Medicine Clinical Terms* (SNOMED CT) in 2002, which combined the College of American Pathologists' *Systematized Nomenclature of Medicine Reference Terminology* with the United Kingdom's National Health Service Clinical Terms Version 3 (previously known as the Read Codes) (116,117). SNOMED CT is described as a computer-compatible medical terminology that provides a basis for accurate translation from medical language into codes for many purposes. It is multilingual and comprises concepts as well as descriptions and information on relationships between concepts. Each concept, description, and relationship has a SNOMED identifier that may have up to 18 digits. It is preferred that each concept in the vocabulary be clearly definable and distinct from all other concepts in the vocabulary. SNOMED's purposes include serving as a means for representing clinical information for consistent and reliable storage and retrieval and improving the quality of health care (118,119).

The road to an international nomenclature of diseases has been a long one. Because of the diverse background and training of physicians practicing all over the world, and because of the different specialties and disciplines in medicine, preparing a list of approved terminology and definitions is difficult. Standardizing medical terminology is an important step toward achieving comparability of statistics on causes of illness and causes of death. However, the degree of specificity and multiple hierarchical structure in a nomenclature are two aspects that make it less useful for statistical purposes, which are better served by a statistical classification. Mapping between SNOMED and ICD is an ongoing project (http://www.ihtsdo.org/) to address this need.

International Classification of Functioning, Disability and Health

The *International Classification of Functioning, Disability and Health* (ICF), recommended for testing at the time of the Ninth Revision, was published by WHO on November 15, 2001, after 7 years of developmental work to ensure that ICF is applicable across cultures, age groups, and genders. Effective in 2001, the new classification was accepted as the international standard to describe and measure health and disability. While ICD provides a classification for the traditional health indicators of causes of illness and death, the ICF focus is on the nature of disabilities and handicaps, and how the social and physical environments affect a person's functioning. ICF is available in the official languages of WHO. Additional information on ICF is available from the NCHS website at: http://www.cdc.gov/nchs/icd.htm.

Nonstatistical uses of multiple-cause data

Multiple-cause files can also be used effectively to identify records that merit special study, including preselected combinations of conditions. Such studies were far more difficult prior to the advent of routine multiple-cause data. For example, to assist in the identification of death records for epidemiological studies, the Registrar-General's Office of England and Wales assigned a 1-digit code to disease entities such as cancer and cardiovascular diseases to identify deaths associated with a limited number of diseases not coded as the underlying cause of death (76). For the United States, the routine availability of multiple-cause data makes it possible to single out certificates with any combination of reported conditions.

| 53 |

CHAPTER 8

Issues Associated With ICD Development

ICD has evolved and grown in complexity as a reflection of changes in medical science, technology, society, and applications of the classification. Two major forces that have contributed to the evolution of ICD are 1) use of the classification for nonstatistical purposes and 2) the effect of automation. These forces, among others, have raised a number of issues for ICD. They include the divergent classification interests of the statistical and nonstatistical communities, the consequences of frequent ICD updates necessitated by nonstatistical uses of the classification, the role of WHO in the revision process, and the impact of automation on the classification. A number of these issues were discussed by Rosenberg at the 2002 Brisbane meeting of the heads of Collaborating Centers (120).

Divergent classification needs of statistical, nonstatistical communities

Shortly after the introduction of ICD–6, the shortcomings of ICD for nonstatistical purposes were becoming ever more apparent to users of that community with respect to the level of detail and frequency of needed updates. The revision conferences prior to the Tenth showed ambivalence with respect to various proposals on adapting ICD for nonstatistical purposes such as indexing hospital charts and medical reimbursement. The ambivalence appears to have been resolved in ICD–10, which cautions users that the revision is not designed for nonstatistical purposes: "[ICD] is neither intended nor suitable for indexing of distinct clinical entities. There are also some constraints on the use of ICD for studies of financial aspects, such as billing or resource allocation" (121). This statement underscores the bedrock principle of ICD as a statistical classification, yet it contradicts manifest developments during the past 50 years which have seen the classification increasingly used for nonstatistical purposes—which in turn have substantially influenced the content of the revisions, especially the level of detail. As of ICD–10, the number of rubrics is many times greater than that of ICD–7, so that the grouping of diseases and conditions in ICD–10 may no longer be suitable for

hospital use. To test the suitability of ICD–10 for indexing hospital charts, a study could be undertaken replicating that carried out in 1959 by AHA and the American Association of Medical Record Librarians.

Up to and including ICD–6, the ICD revision process was relatively simple. The ever-increasing detail of ICD has added to the complexity of the classification. Until ICD–9, ICD was basically a classification for the compilation of statistics on causes of illness and causes of death. In ICD–9, proposals from a number of medical specialties were incorporated. In ICD–10, the needs of more medical specialties were accommodated. Meeting the needs of specialists has complicated the revision process. The uses proposed by and the orientation of the various medical specialties differ greatly, which makes it difficult to maintain a consistent axis of classification throughout ICD. The amount of detail required by specialists usually exceeds the needs for general use. In addition, the sophistication of specialists often leads to fine distinctions not readily recognized in general medical practice. Many of the clinical modifications of ICD–9–CM also found their way into ICD–10.

At the time of the Eighth Revision, Dorn saw difficulties arising from the efforts to utilize ICD for multiple purposes. In a paper prepared for the Subcommittee on International List Revision, a subcommittee of the U.S. National Committee on Vital and Health Statistics that he chaired, Dorn called attention to the dominant role of mortality uses of ICD despite its increasing use for the classification and coding of morbidity statistics and for indexing hospital records (122).

Dorn felt that the time had come "for squarely facing the question, can the International Statistical Classification be successfully used for these three purposes, that is, for mortality statistics, for morbidity statistics, and for indexing hospital records?" He expressed his belief that the preparation of a single disease classification for multiple purposes can be greatly simplified if two essential steps were kept in mind. These were 1) the construction of a classified list of diagnoses, and 2) the development of principles and procedures for using this classification for indexing records and for coding and tabulating morbidity and mortality statistics. The situation with respect to uses of ICD has changed considerably from the time of Dorn. Mortality uses no longer appear to dominate ICD or its uses—nonstatistical uses do.

Thus, the needs of morbidity—a relative latecomer to ICD uses—have assumed an increasingly important role in structuring the ICD process as well as ICD content. This has led to a dichotomy within the ICD user community, specifically between those who use ICD for statistical applications and those who use ICD for nonstatistical applications. The statistical users, principally mortality data users, need continuity for trend analysis rather than frequent updates, and broad levels of disease aggregation consistent with diagnostic reporting on death certificates. In contrast, the administrative users need the most up-to-date diagnostic terminology and entity specificity.

Frequent updates in ICD impose a heavy burden on mortality data users because the statistical impact of any changes in ICD must be measured to determine the quantitative impact on trends and patterns in mortality. Revisions, therefore, must be accompanied by bridge-coding or comparability studies. In addition, classification changes have implications for tabulation lists—that is, the list of diseases used in tabular presentations. And, critically, revisions require changes in coding procedures, coding training, and their automated, electronic counterparts—the computer programs that automatically generate multiple or underlying causes of death. Together—changes in tabulation lists, coding training, revisions in computer programs, and revisions in tabulation lists and publications—impose enormous costs in terms of dollars and human resources.

Thus, the requirements of nonstatistical users, especially in a health services setting, place an enormous burden on the statistical user community. It would be fair to say that the perspectives and needs of mortality and morbidity users of ICD and those of health administrators have diverged, and that increasingly the ICD process is propelled by administrative rather than statistical and research needs.

Consequences of frequent updating

The annual updating process has been implemented through the active functioning of the Mortality Reference Group, the Update and Revision Committee, and decisions ratified by the center heads at annual meetings since 1997. However, a number of process issues such as dissemination of updates have taken longer to resolve (43). For example, as of 2003, many of the changes had not been disseminated by WHO in either electronic form on the WHO-ICD

website, or in published form, but the changes had been incorporated into the ACME software used by a number of countries for producing annual mortality files. Uneven implementation of ICD changes resulting from the ICD continuous updating process consequently can produce noncomparable mortality statistics between countries.

The continuous updating process naturally raises questions that have implications for the process of developing another major revision, that is, an Eleventh Revision (ICD–11). Because developing and implementing a new revision have enormous costs for both WHO and the member nations, the updating process may ease some needs for revision as well as illuminate logistic questions that need to be addressed.

Role of WHO in revision process

The role of WHO and its predecessor organizations in the ICD revision process has changed over time. The apparent shift in responsibility for the revision of ICD from the Expert Committee on Health Statistics to WHO center heads undoubtedly facilitated the revision process because it more or less kept the preparatory work within the WHO family. The center heads were bound by a common purpose and interest, and there was no need to educate the group on the objectives or the revision process.

The preparatory work for ICD–11 broadens input, as anyone can submit proposals (http://extranet.who.int/icdrevision). However, topical work groups play a key role in developing proposals and considering proposals submitted by other parties.

Automation

Computer technology has great implications for ICD. The potential and manifest applications extend all the way from information capture at the basic record level, through data processing, to data analysis, and dissemination. In each of these areas, important strides have already been made and portend even greater and improved applications in the future, with implications that are difficult to predict but, on the whole, are likely to be favorable to uniformity, accuracy, and timeliness for both mortality and morbidity applications.

Data capture

Electronic data capture, particularly for mortality, raises the question of who will enter the data into the electronic death registration systems? ICD recommendation and regulation has dictated that the medical certification of death be completed by a medical professional, preferably the certifying physician. In an electronic environment, will this continue? Or will the function be delegated to a medical records management specialist who has had no direct experience with the course of the disease that led to death, and who will not be able to benefit from the interactive functions of electronic systems, including online queries, edits, and tutorials?

A second question in relation to data capture is whether electronic registration systems will, by virtue of their simplicity, incorporate predetermined, fixed lists of diagnoses from which the certifier makes a selection, or whether an open format—which is highly preferred and required by ICD—be maintained. An open format allows the certifier to use his or her own words and style of medical certification; a fixed list has the danger of limiting medical terminology, nuance, detail, and change.

Data processing

Capabilities of capturing literal diagnostic language, or using codes (such as the SuperMICAR ERNs) that are more detailed than ICD categories, have the potential of eventually supplanting ICD for some statistical and nonstatistical purposes. Data users are likely to be interested in more rather than less detailed diagnostic information if it can be retrieved from a database, especially if the more detailed categories can be collapsed into categories that are consistent with ICD and other classification systems. The analytical potential use for using ERNs should be recognized and examined.

Automation has major consequences for the profession of medical coding, as recognized and discussed in detail at the International Collaborative Effort on Automating Mortality (ICE)—a conference first sponsored by NCHS in 1996 (123), and again in 1999 and 2003 (57,124).

The introduction of automation drastically alters the nature of jobs that previously produced the outputs on a manual basis. In the case of mortality medical coding, automation has had the expected effects: productivity, accuracy, and comparability of coding are greatly increased, and, consequently, far fewer manual coders are needed to accomplish the same tasks.

One of the automation issues, therefore, is what types of mortality medical coding expertise will be required in an automated environment? The ICE conferences concluded that coders will still be needed, but far fewer and with higher levels of skills than previously. Although coders for the most part will not be involved in production, in small numbers they will be needed to provide coding solutions to problems that cannot be handled by the automated systems arising from new diseases, changed etiological relationships, new categories, periodic ICD modifications,

and technical assistance needs of analysts and researchers. Highly skilled coders will also be needed for quality control of the automated systems, where small systematic samples will be manually coded to ensure that cause-of-death assignments are consistent between automated and manual systems.

Recruiting and retaining mortality medical coders has always been a challenge but will be even more formidable given the high-order qualifications needed to work in an automated environment. Through its Education Committee, WHO, and WHO Collaborating Centers for the Family of International Classification are addressing the issues of credentialing medical coders to enhance their professional status and to improve the attractiveness of these essential jobs in automated environments.

Data dissemination

Automation makes possible the ready dissemination of ICD and its related products through the Internet, to which most of the world now has access. Theoretically, ICD and its latest updates can be made available almost immediately to the universe of classification users. The most complex issues that arise are not dissimilar to those currently associated with other products heretofore available in nonelectronic media, such as music, books, newspapers, and journals. The issues have to do with ownership and costs—many of these products are produced on the assumption that they will generate some revenue to cover production costs. To some degree, similar issues have arisen over the years in connection with ICD, in particular regarding the rights to adapt it, in national versions, for medical reimbursement purposes. WHO must consider how best to take advantage of electronic capabilities in the furtherance of public health without jeopardizing its financial situation and ownership rights.

CHAPTER 9
Summary

This report traces related and sometimes intertwining efforts, particularly those leading toward the development of nomenclatures, death registration, and most importantly for this report, disease classification. An essential step in using information on records of illness or death is converting the reported diagnostic information into codes that can be used for statistical tabulation and analysis. The conversion is accomplished using a disease classification in which diagnostic entities have unique codes. In the case of causes of death, such a classification system is known by the operational name *International Classification of Diseases* (ICD). For over 100 years, ICD has stood as a major achievement of international statistical cooperation for public health. It is regarded as the authoritative classification for causes of death and illness and is available in the official languages of the United Nations—English, French, Spanish, Russian, and Chinese—as well as in various other languages. Over time, ICD has become increasingly detailed and complex, and its uses have gone well beyond its original intent: a classification conceived to classify causes of death for statistical tabulation and research. The classification is increasingly used for nonstatistical purposes, initially for medical records indexing and increasingly now for medical reimbursement. This change in emphasis has affected the content of the classification and, recently, the updating process. Adaptations have also been made for use by various medical specialties, and in a growing number of countries including the United States, a clinical modification of ICD is in use to meet the needs of nonstatistical ICD users.

The classification includes a medical certificate form and rules for selecting the cause of death for mortality tabulations that still reflect those proposed by Bertillon in ICD–1. Up to ICD–6, the international medical certificate form and coding rules served as models for countries to follow. However, countries adopted whatever suited their interest and convenience. This casual attitude toward international comparability changed after the Sixth Revision Conference when WHO Regulations No.1 came into effect. The provisions of these regulations are as binding upon countries as any international treaty. In effect, official mortality statistics on causes of death are derived from the medical certification of causes of death prepared by the physician in attendance at the time of death using the medical certificate form from the classification.

The international rules for classifying the cause of death for mortality tabulations are subject to modification at the time of ICD revision and, beginning with ICD–10, annually. Most of the modifications that have been made represent clarification of old rules or additions to cope with new problems. Occasionally, significant substantive changes have been made such as when the international rules for selecting the underlying cause of death were adopted as part of ICD–6.

Major revisions of the classification of diseases and of coding rules produce discontinuities in mortality trends of causes of death, which need to be considered in any comparison of data between two periods of time or between two countries. The effect of such breaks may be studied by what has been termed "bridge coding," that is, the classification of data for the same period of years by the new and old classification of diseases and coding procedures. Comparability ratios derived from such a study provide a measure of revision changes. A major advance in mortality statistics was the introduction of automated coding in the United States, a development that has spread to other countries, many of which have adopted the same software. This development has many benefits, including improving comparability and consistency.

An enduring concern of vital statistics, epidemiologists, and the public health community is the quality of cause-of-death statistics. Studies have been made using as the basis of comparison various sources of data such as postmortem examinations, hospital and physician records, and all sources of medical information. The precise measurement of the accuracy and completeness of reporting cause-of-death information is not possible. However, there is little question that improvement in the quality of medical certification is desirable as a continuing goal. A variety of methods for improving medical certification are available.

Despite the recognized limitations of primary, or single-cause, mortality tabulations, they have served well the purposes for which they were intended. Multiple-cause statistics were produced periodically in the United States until automated coding made possible annual production, effective with the 1968 data year, to address some concerns with single-cause tabulations. However, multiple-cause data cannot fully address the concerns because these data are making use of supplemental information from a form designed to capture the single underlying cause.

The increasing influence of nonstatistical uses and automation present a number of challenges to the maintenance and development of ICD. These challenges will no doubt be met through continuing international collaboration and cooperation, under the aegis of WHO.

| 60 |

References

1. Graunt J. Natural and political observations in a following index and made upon the bills of mortality. London. 1662.

2. Eyler J. Victorian social medicine: The ideas and methods of William Farr. Baltimore: Johns Hopkins University Press. 1979.

3. Pelling M. Cholera, fever, and English medicine, 1825–1865. Oxford Press; p. 92–102. 1978.

4. Hetzel AM. History and organization of the vital statistics system. Hyattsville, MD: National Center for Health Statistics. 1997.

5. Registrar General of England and Wales. First annual report of the registrar-general of births, deaths, and marriages in England. London: His Majesty's Stationery Office; p. 99–102. 1839.

6. Robb-Smith AHT. A history of the college's nomenclature of diseases: Its preparation. Journal of the Royal College of Physicians 3(4):341–58. London. 1969.

7. Robb-Smith AHT. A history of the college's nomenclature of diseases: Its reception. Journal of the Royal College of Physicians 4(1):5–26. London. 1969.

8. American Medical Association. Standard nomenclature of diseases and operations. 5th ed. Thompson ET, Hayden AC, eds. New York: McGraw-Hill. 1961.

9. Logie HB. A standard classified nomenclature of diseases. New York: The Commonwealth Fund. 1933.

10. Webster's dictionary. 7th ed. 1972.

11. U.S. Bureau of the Census. Standard nomenclature of diseases, pathological conditions, injuries, and poisonings for the United States. Davis WH, ed. Washington, DC: Government Printing Office. 1920.

12. American Medical Association. Current medical terminology. Gordon BL, ed. Chicago. 1963.

13. American Medical Association. Current medical information and terminology. 4th ed. Gordon BL, editor. Chicago. 1971.

14. American Medical Association. Current medical information and terminology (CMIT). 5th ed. Finkel AJ, editor. Chicago. 1981.

15. American Medical Association. Current procedural terminology. Gordon BL, ed. Chicago. 1966.

16. American Medical Association. Physicians' current procedural terminology. Gordon BL, ed. Chicago. 1984.

17. World Health Organization. International statistical classification of diseases and related health problems, ICD–10. Vol. 1. Geneva. 1992.

18. Cullen W. Synopsis of nosology (translated from Latin by John Thompson). Philadelphia: Thomas Dobson. 1816.

19. International Statistical Institute. Proceedings of the Meeting in Kristiana, 1899, Vol II, Part I.

20. U.S. Bureau of the Census. Manual of international classification of causes of death. Adopted by the U.S. Census Office for the compilation of mortality statistics, for use beginning with the year 1900. Washington, DC: Government Printing Office. 1901.

21. U.S. Bureau of the Census. Manual of the international list of causes of death. Based on the second decennial revision by the international commission, Paris, July 1 to 3, 1909. Washington, DC: Government Printing Office. 1909.

22. U.S. Bureau of the Census. Manual of the international list of causes of death. Based on the third decennial revision by the international commission, Paris, October 11 to 15, 1920. Washington, DC: Government Printing Office. 1924.

23. U.S. Bureau of the Census. Manual of the international list of causes of death. Based on the fourth decennial revision by the international commission, Paris, October 16 to 19, 1929. Washington, DC: Government Printing Office. 1931.

24. U.S. Bureau of the Census. Manual of the international list of causes of death (fifth revision) and joint causes of death (fourth edition). Washington, DC: Government Printing Office. 1939.

25. Dominion Council of Health of Canada. A standard morbidity code. 1936.

26. U.S. Public Health Service. Manual for coding causes of illness. Misc. Pub. No. 32. Washington, DC: U.S. Government Printing Office. 1944.

27. Medical Research Council. A provisional classification of diseases and injuries for use in compiling morbidity statistics. Special Report Series No. 248. London: His Majesty's Stationery Office. 1944.

28. World Health Organization. Manual of the international statistical classification of diseases,

injuries, and causes of death. Sixth revision of the international lists of diseases and causes of death. Adopted 1948. Geneva. 1948.

29. World Health Organization. Report of the international conference for the seventh revision of the international lists of diseases and causes of death, Paris, April 21–26, 1955. WHO/HS/7Rev.Conf.17/Rev.1. Geneva. 1955.

30. World Health Organization. Manual of the international statistical classification of diseases, injuries, and causes of death. Based on the recommendations of the seventh revision conference, 1955, and adopted by the ninth World Health Assembly under the WHO nomenclature regulations. Geneva. 1957.

31. World Health Organization. Report of the international conference for the eighth revision of the international classification of diseases, July 6–12, 1965. WHO/HS/8 Rev. Conf./11/65. Geneva. 1965.

32. World Health Organization. Manual of the international statistical classification of diseases, injuries, and causes of death. Based on recommendations of the eighth revision conference, 1965, and adopted by the nineteenth World Health Assembly. Geneva. 1967.

33. World Health Organization. Report of the international conference for the ninth revision of the international classification of diseases, September 30–October 6, 1975. WHO/ICD9/Rev.Conf./75.24. Geneva. 1976.

34. World Health Organization. Manual of the international classification of diseases, injuries, and causes of death, based on the recommendations of the ninth revision conference, 1975, and adopted by the twenty-ninth World Health Assembly. Geneva. 1977.

35. American Psychiatric Association, Committee on Nomenclature and Statistics. Diagnostic and statistical manual of mental disorders. 2nd ed. Washington, DC. 1968.

36. World Health Organization. International statistical classification of impairments, disabilities and handicaps. Geneva. 1980.

37. World Health Organization. International classification of diseases for oncology. 1st ed. Geneva. 1976.

38. World Health Organization. International classification of diseases for oncology. 2nd ed. Percy C, Holden V, Muir C, eds. Geneva. 1990.

39. Percy C. Cancer data systems VI. Alteration of cancer statistics by the 8th and 9th revisions of the international classification of diseases. Curr Probl Cancer IX(3):61–77. 1985.

40. American Academy of Opthalmology and Otolaryngology. International nomenclature of opthalmology. Rochester, MN. 1977.

41. World Health Organization. Report of the international conference for the tenth revision of the international classification of diseases, September 26–October 2, 1989. Geneva. 1986. Available from: WHO/ICD10/Rev. Conf./89.19.

42. World Health Organization. Report of the meeting of heads of WHO collaborating centres for the classification of diseases, Copenhagen, Denmark, October 14–20, 1997. WHO/HST/ICD/C/97.65 and http://www.who.int/classifications/network/en/cophenagen.pdf.

43. World Health Organization. WHO/GPE/CAS/C/01.32. Bethesda, MD. 2001.

44. Twain M. The adventures of Huckleberry Finn. Chapter XVIII; p. 185–6. Bantam Classic. 1988.

45. Humphreys NA. Vital statistics: Memorial volume of selections from the reports and writings of William Farr. London: Offices of the Sanitary Institute. 1885.

46. Pearl R. Introduction to medical biometry and statistics. New York: W.B. Saunders Company; p. 64. 1940.

47. DePorte JV. Mortality statistics and the physician. Am J Public Health 31(10):1051–6. 1941.

48. Tolson GC, Barnes JM, Gay GA, Kowaleski JL. The 1989 revision of the U.S. standard certificates and reports. Vital Health Stat 4(28). Hyattsville, MD: National Center for Health Statistics. 1991.

49. International Statistical Institute. Proceedings of the First Congress. Brussels. 1853.

50. U.S. Bureau of the Census. Index of joint causes of death. Printed in proof. 1914.

51. U.S. Bureau of the Census. Manual of joint causes of death. Washington, DC: U.S. Government Printing Office. 1925.

52. U.S. Bureau of the Census. Manual of joint causes of death. Washington, DC: U.S. Government Printing Office. 1935.

53. Green D. Preliminary findings on study of the rules for underlying cause of death. ICD/C/82.16. Caracus, Venezuela: World Health Organization. 1982.

54. Anderson RN, Minino AM, Hoyert DL, Rosenberg HM. Comparability of cause of death between ICD–9 and ICD–10: Preliminary estimates. National vital statistics reports; vol 49, no 2. Hyattsville, MD: National Center for Health Statistics. 2001.

55. World Health Organization. WHO long-term strategy for the development and management of health-related classifications. WHO/HST/ICD/C/97.39 and http://whqlibdoc.who.int/hq/1997/WHO_HST_ICD_C_97.39_REV.1.pdf. Copenhagen, Denmark. 1997.

56. Rosenberg HM. Overview of the NCHS systems. Proceedings of the International Collaborative Effort on Automating Mortality Statistics, Volume II. Minino AM, Rosenberg HM, eds. Hyattsville, MD: National Center for Health Statistics. 2001.

57. National Center for Health Statistics. Proceedings of the International Collaborative Effort on Automating Mortality Statistics, Volume II. Minino AM, Rosenberg HM, eds. Hyattsville, MD. 2001. Available from: http://www.cdc.gov/nchs/data/misc/ice01_acc.pdf.

58. Eurostat. Roadmap for causes of death, 2008. Available from: http://circa.europa.eu/Public/irc/dsis/health/library?l=/methodologiessandsdatasc/causessofsdeath/road_causes_death&vm=detailed&sb=Title. Accessed November 1, 2010.

59. Chamblee RF, Evans MC, Rosenberg HM. A national multiple cause statistical system. Proceedings of the Social Statistics Section, American Statistical Association; p.13–5. 1979.

60. National Center for Health Statistics. Instructions for classifying multiple causes of death. NCHS instruction manual; part 2B. Hyattsville, MD: Public Health Service. Published annually.

61. Johansson LA, G Pavillon. IRIS: A language-independent coding system based on the NCHS system MMDS. WHO-FIC Network Meeting. Tokyo. 2005.

62. Biraud Y. A method of recording of crude causes of death by laymen in underdeveloped countries. African Conference on Vital and Health Statistics. November 19–24, 1956. CCTA/WHO/STATS CONF.7.

63. World Health Organization. Lay reporting of health information. Geneva. 1978.

64. Lukovic G, Ivancovic D. Development of cause of death data and deaths without medical attention. Final report of the methodological study and annex to the final report on the methodological study [unpublished]. Zagreb, Yugoslavia: Medical School, Andrija Stampar School of Public Health, University of Zagreb. 1978.

65. Chandramohan D, Maurde GH, Rodrigues LD, Hayes RJ. Verbal autopsies for adult deaths: Issues in their development and validation. Int J Epidemiol 23(2):213–22. 1994.

66. World Health Organization. Verbal autopsy standards: Ascertaining and attributing cause of death. Geneva. 2007.

67. Chamblee RF, Evans MC. TRANSAX, the NCHS system for producing multiple cause-of-death statistics, 1968–78. Vital Health Stat 1(20). National Center for Health Statistics. Washington, DC: U.S. Government Printing Office. 1986.

68. National Center for Health Statistics. Vital statistics, ICD–9 TRANSAX disease reference tables for classifying multiple causes of death. NCHS instruction manual, part 2F. Hyattsville, MD. Published annually.

69. National Center for Health Statistics. Public use data file documentation: Multiple cause of death for ICD–9 1993 data. Hyattsville, MD. 1995.

70. National Center for Health Statistics. National Mortality Followback Survey, 1996, documentation. Available from: http://www.cdc.gov/nchs/nvss/nmfs.htm.

71. Dorn HF, Moriyama IM. Uses and significance of multiple cause tabulations for mortality statistics. Am J Public Health 54(3):400–6. 1964.

72. National Center for Health Statistics. ICD–9 underlying cause-of-death lists for tabulating mortality statistics (1979), vital statistics instruction manual, part 9. Hyattsville, MD. 1979.

73. Israel RA. Some considerations regarding the presentation of multiple cause data. ICD/MC/69.7. Geneva: World Health Organization. 1969.

74. Hanzlick R, ed. The medical cause of death manual. Chicago: College of American Pathologists. 1994.

75. Kochanek KD, Rosenberg HM. Issues, considerations and examples in the use of multiple cause data in United States government statistics. WHO Heads of Collaborating Centers' Ad Hoc Meeting on Multiple Cause Analysis. London. April 1994.

76. Adelstein A. Multiple cause analysis. WHO/ICD/Rev. Conf./75.16. Geneva: World Health Organization. 1975.

77. National Center for Health Statistics. Multiple causes of death in the United States. Monthly vital statistics report; vol 32 no 10 (Suppl 2). Hyattsville, MD. 1984.

78. Israel RA, Rosenberg HM, Curtin LR. Analytical potential for multiple cause-of-death data. Am J Epidemiol 124(2):161–79. 1986.

79. World Health Organization. Comparison of cause-of-death coding: Canada, England, and Wales, and the United States of America. WHO/HS/Nat.Com./114. Geneva: WHO Classification Center. 1958.

80. World Health Organization. Studies on the accuracy and comparability of statistics on causes of death. EURO 215.1/16. Copenhagen: WHO Regional Office for Europe. 1966.

81. World Health Organization. Medical certification of causes of death: Report of a study. Copenhagen: WHO Regional Office for Europe. 1973.

82. Registrar-General of England and Wales. The Registrar-General's statistical review of England and Wales for the years 1938 and 1939. London: His Majesty's Stationery Office. 1947.

83. Dunn HL, Shackley W. Comparison of cause-of-death assignments by the 1929 and 1938 revisions of the international list: Deaths in the United States, 1940. National Office of Vital Statistics. Vital statistics–special reports; vol 19 no 14. Washington, DC: U.S. Government Printing Office. 1944.

84. Faust MM, Dolman AB. Comparability ratios based on mortality statistics for the fifth and sixth revisions: United States, 1950. National Office of Vital Statistics. Vital statistics–special reports; vol 51 no 3; p. 135–62. Washington, DC: U.S. Government Printing Office. 1964.

85. Faust MM, Dolman AB. Comparability of mortality statistics for the sixth and seventh revisions: United States, 1958. Vital statistics–special reports; vol 51 no 4; p. 248–97. National Office of Vital Statistics. Washington, DC: U.S. Government Printing Office. 1965.

86. Klebba AJ. Provisional estimates of selected comparability ratios based on dual coding of 1966 death certificates by the seventh and eighth revisions of the international classification of diseases. National Center for Health Statistics. Monthly vital statistics report; vol 17 no 8 (Suppl). Washington, DC. 1968.

87. Klebba AJ. Estimates of selected comparability ratios based on dual coding of 1976 death certificates by the eighth and ninth revisions of the international classification of diseases. Monthly vital statistics report; vol 25 no 11 (Suppl). Hyattsville, MD: National Center for Health Statistics. 1980.

88. Rooney C. Comparability issues and bridge coding methods. In Arialdi M, Rosenberg HM, editors. Proceedings of the International Collaborative Effort on Automating Mortality Statistics, vol II; p. 145–8. Hyattsville, MD: National Center for Health Statistics. 2001.

89. Greig M, Walker S. The effect of changing from manual to automated coding. In Arialdi M, Rosenberg HM, editors. Proceedings of the International Collaborative Effort on Automating Mortality Statistics, vol II; p. 287–92. Hyattsville, MD. 2001.

90. Hoyert DL, Arias E, Smith BL, et al. Deaths: Final data for 1999. National vital statistics reports; vol 49 no 8. Hyattsville, MD: National Center for Health Statistics. 2001.

91. Rosenberg HM. Cause of death as a contemporary problem. J Hist Med Allied Sci 54:133–53. 1999.

92. National Center for Health Statistics. Vital statistics of the United States, vol. II, mortality, part A, 1977. Technical appendix. Washington, DC: U.S. Government Printing Office. 1981.

93. Modan B, Wagener DK, Feldman JJ, Rosenberg HM, Feinleib M. Increased mortality from brain tumors: A combined outcome of diagnostic technology and change of attitude toward the elderly. Am J Epidemiol 135(2):1349–57. 1992.

94. Hoyert DL, Rosenberg HM, MacDorman MF. Effect of changes in death certificate format on cause-specific mortality trends, United States, 1979–1992. Death certification and mortality statistics: An international perspective. Coleman MP, Aylin P, editors. Studies on medical and population subjects No. 64. London: Her Majesty's Stationery Office; p. 47–58. 2000.

95. Gittlesohn A, Royston P. Annotated bibliography of cause-of-death validation studies: 1958–1980. Vital Health Stat 2(89). Hyattsville, MD: National Center for Health Statistics. 1982.

96. Rosenberg HM. The nature and accuracy of cause-of-death data. Report of the Workshop on Improving Cause-of-Death Statistics. Appendix p. 1–5. Hyattsville, MD: National Center for Health Statistics and National Committee on Vital and Health Statistics. 1989.

97. Berkson J. Limitations of the application of four-fold table analysis to hospital data. Biometrics Bulletin 2:47. 1946.

98. Mainland D. The risk of fallacious conclusions from autopsy data on the incidence of disease with application to heart disease. Am Heart J 45:644. 1953.

99. Cornfield J. Principles of research. American Journal of Mental Deficiency 64:240. 1959.

100. Rosenberg HM. The impact of cause-of-death querying. Report of the workshop on improving cause-of-death statistics. Appendix p. 1–14. Hyattsville, MD: National Center for Health Statistics and National Committee on Vital and Health Statistics. 1989.

101. Hoyert DL, Lima A. Querying of death certificates in the United States. Public Health Rep 120. 2005.

102. National Center for Health Statistics. Cause-of-death querying manual. Vital statistics instruction manual, part 20. Hyattsville, MD. 2007.

103. Rip-Botha CM, Wood M. The effect of query action on coded mortality data: An Australian study. In Arialdi M, Rosenberg HM, eds. Proceedings of the International Collaborative Effort on Automating Mortality Statistics, vol II; p. 88–95. Hyattsville, MD: National Center for Health Statistics. 2001.

104. National Center for Health Statistics and U.S. National Committee on Vital and Health Statistics. Report of the workshop on improving cause-of-death statistics, Virginia Beach, Virginia, October 15–17, 1989. Hyattsville, MD. 1989.

105. National Center for Health Statistics and U.S. National Committee on Vital and Health Statistics. Report of the second workshop on improving cause-of-death statistics, Virginia Beach, Virginia, April 21–23, 1991. Hyattsville, MD. 1991.

106. National Center for Health Statistics. Writing cause-of-death statements. Available from: http://www.cdc.gov/nchs/nvss/writing_cod_statements.htm. Accessed January 12, 2011.

107. National Center for Health Statistics. 2003 revisions of the U.S. Standard Certificates of Live Birth and Death and the Fetal Death Report. Available from: http://www.cdc.gov/nchs/nvss/vital_certificate_revisions.htm.

108. National Center for Health Statistics. Death edit specifications for the 2003 revision of the U.S. Standard Certificate of Death. 2005. Available from: http://www.cdc.gov/nchs/data/dvs/FinalDeathSpecs2-22-05.pdf.

109. Smith AF, Weed JA, Mingay DJ, Jobe JB. The effect of condition sequencing order on cause-of-death statistics. WHO/99.26. Geneva: World Health Organization. 1999.

110. American Hospital Association. Efficiency of the coding system of the international classification of diseases and standard nomenclature of diseases. Journal of the American Association of Medical Records Librarians 30(3). 1959.

111. U.S. Public Health Service. The international classification of diseases, adapted for indexing hospital records by diseases and operations. Public health service publication; no 719 (rev). Washington, DC: U.S. Government Printing Office. 1962.

112. U.S. Public Health Service. Eighth revision international classification of diseases adapted for use in the United States. Public health service publication; no 1693. Washington, DC: U.S. Government Printing Office. 1967.

113. National Center for Health Statistics and Health Care Financing Administration. International classification of diseases, ninth revision, clinical modification, ICD-CM, fourth edition. Washington, DC: U.S. Government Printing Office. 1991.

114. College of American Pathologists. Systematized nomenclature of medicine (SNOMED). 1st ed. Skokie, IL. 1965.

115. College of American Pathologists. Systematized nomenclature of medicine (SNOMED). 2nd ed. Cote R, ed. Skokie, IL. 1979.

116. International Health Terminology Standards Development Organisation. History of SNOMED CT. Available from: http://www.ihtsdo.org/snomed-ct/history0/. Accessed October 1, 2009.

117. College of American Pathologists. SNOMED historical perspectives. Available from: http://www.cap.org/apps/cap.portal?_nfpb=true&cntvwrPtlt_actionOverride=%2Fportlets%2FcontentViewer%2Fshow&_windowLabel=cntvwrPtlt&cntvwrPtlt%7BactionForm.contentReference%7D=snomed%2FhistPersp.html&_state=maximized&_pageLabel=cntvwr. Accessed October 1, 2009.

118. Imel M. A closer look: The SNOMED clinical terms to ICD–9–CM mapping. J AHIMA 73(6):66–9. 2002.

119. International Health Terminology Standards Development Organisation. SNOMED CT style guide: Introduction and overview. Purpose, scope, boundaries, and requirements. Version 0.01. 2008. Available from: http://www.ihtsdo.org/fileadmin/user_upload/Docs_01/Copenhagen_Apr_2008/SNOMED_CT_Style_Guides/IHTSDO_Modeling_StyleGuide-Overview-20080408_v0-01.pdf. Accessed October 1, 2009.

120. Rosenberg HM. Approaches to implementing ICD–10 for vital statistics. WHO/GPE/CAS/C/01.01. Brisbane, Australia, October 14–19, 2002.

121. World Health Organization. International statistical classification of diseases and related health problems, tenth revision. Instruction manual 2:2. Geneva. 1993.

122. Dorn HF. Some considerations in the revision of the international statistical classification. Public Health Rep 79(2):175–9. 1964.

123. National Center for Health Statistics. Proceedings of the International Collaborative Effort on Automating Mortality Statistics, Volume I. Peters K, ed. Hyattsville, MD. 1999. Available from: http://www.cdc.gov/nchs/data/misc/ice99_1.pdf.

124. National Center for Health Statistics. Proceedings of the International Collaborative Effort on Automating Mortality Statistics, Volume III. Minino AM, Rosenberg HM, eds. Hyattsville, MD. 2006. Available from: http://www.cdc.gov/nchs/data/misc/ice06_3.pdf.